What Others Are Saying

I need Anastasia to earn $$$

"Before I started working with Anastasia, my body had shut down as a result of 6 car accidents over several years. My brain was foggy, I had no energy, I couldn't deliver speeches coherently, I was in pain, and I could barely earn money. Within the first month, my brain started working again, my pain vanished and my energy skyrocketed. During the six months I've been working with Anastasia, I have earned an average of $10,000 per month. I took a month hiatus and realized I needed to continue working with her because she does something special with my brain that no other health practitioner has been able to do, and I have been to many."
— **Dr. Marion Mehrer, Executive Placement Services**

Helped when no one else could, instantly uplifting:

"Anastasia is THE MOST AMAZING INTUITIVE ENERGY HEALER I've ever met! She helped me when no one else could. Truly not of this world. Fascinating, extremely accurate & instantly uplifting, I promise— you will never feel the same again! Unblock, Clear & Attract —Go See Her!! "
——**Cindy Goldenberg, TV Personality and Medium at** CindyGoldenberg.com

Vertigo cleared fast:

"Anastasia really helped me when I had a lingering case of vertigo and could no longer function. One session and the vertigo was gone! I love when she is around, I always feel better."
— **Marcia Weider, Founder of DreamUniversity.com**

Energy and Vitality Significantly Increased:

"Dr. Anastasia Chopelas is the person I recommend to all my colleagues who need healing and traditional medicine or practices have failed. Her message needs to be heard. Anastasia has been my healer and I've noticed my energy and vitality significantly increase."
Eiji Morishita, Founder of Speak Your Genius

Banished 40 years of fatigue:

"While I was speaking to Anastasia on the phone, my hands began tingling. After the half-hour consultation, I got off the phone and my energy levels climbed so much. For many years, I have suffered from fatigue and needed to sleep long hours. I have tried everything and everyone. In the weeks after our session, I haven't needed to sleep as much and I have had so much more energy than I've felt in years."
—-Amanda Kent, Financial Advisor

Cleared sore throat at critical event almost instantly:
"One of the people I met on the Marketer's Cruise dinner was Anastasia. She really helped me out. This was the first day of the cruise and I had already lost my voice. This was the beginning of a seven day adventure where I had to meet and greet, and talk to lots of people and I couldn't speak. Literally, within a half an hour of meeting her and she doing her amazing healing work on me, my voice returned. By the time dinner was over that night, my voice was fully back and I was able to enjoy the cruise. If you have an opportunity to work with her in any capacity, I highly recommend it. It was completely magical what she did for me and I'm sure she'll do the same for you. "
— Teddy Garcia, InfoMarketingSystem.com

Lost sugar cravings, more serene and focused:
"I would recommend Anastasia to anyone who is interested to begin their personal healing process. I found her to be caring and very knowledgeable. After my visit with her I felt more serene and focused, lost my sugar cravings. I noticed increased motivation regarding tasks and projects that needed to be addressed in my life. Her meditation tape is outstanding. I feel that I am now able to do what it takes to accomplish all that I am setting out to do."
—Ellen R. Conejo Valley

Immediate results:
"There a clarity, breadth and understanding in Anastasia's work that lends itself to immediate results and continuous ongoing improvements. She cleared my stubborn lung congestion when no one else could. I give her my highest recommendation."
— Lisa Greenfield, Intuitive at TruthinHand.com

Better clarity, new possibilities:

"Anastasia is incredible. She is a truly gifted healer with a unique approach that is grounded in clear scientific facts that are easy for anyone to understand. Since my session with her, my mind has been clear and I have felt a breath of new possibilities enter my life. I look forward to working with her again and would highly recommend her to anyone looking for clarity or restoration on any level."
— **Sarah Nehamen, InJoyArtistry.com**

One simple tip opens new possibilities:
"When I met Anastasia, she gave me one simple tip. It's totally transformed my life already. I've been doing this one little exercise for just 24 hours, twice. The ideas that are now accessible to me are unbelievable. It really opened me up. I can't wait to work with Anastasia. She's fabulous. You have GOT to check her out."
— **Elaine Starling, Why5PercentSucceed.com**

When no one else could help:
"For the last ten years, I've been seeking help from every kind of healing and medical practitioners I could find that offered hope for my severe and ongoing migraine headaches. Pain medications were just not helping. I went through two surgeries, had my allergies cleared by NAET, cleaned up my environment, and many more things. Nothing helped until I started working with Anastasia. After just two sessions, I started noticing a real difference. After a month, I stopped having headaches except for occasionally. She recorded a special healing audio for me and it really helps when I feel a migraine coming on. Totally dissipates the pain. I have told everyone about her and the incredible help she's given me. I highly recommend her."
— **Tania McComas, Award Winning Hollywood Make up Artist**

The dimension and depth of regained sight is a blessing:
"Anastasia, the work you did with me for my eyes at one of your live trainings was illuminating. I knew that my sight was degenerating and it was of great concern to me. I could feel the changes as I sat there and you worked on clearing my eyes and bringing in regeneration. When I opened them I was astonished to see that there was a pattern on the walls. Before your healing, it looked like a flat solid color. The dimension and depth of regained sight was a blessing."
— **Gwen Lepard, UnreasonableCoach.com**

A Transformational Read:
"This book is such a treasure and so needed... a transformational read that will bring benefit to anyone who has the opportunity to read it. Profound discoveries for anyone seeking to retain or revitalize the wealth of their health!!!"
— **Michele Plunckett, Author of "Innate Wealth: Your Focus, Your Fortune"**

Energy and Vitality Significantly Improve
"Dr. Anastasia Chopelas is the person I recommend to all my colleagues who need healing and traditional medicine or practices have failed. Her message needs to be heard. Anastasia has been my healer and I've noticed my energy and vitality significantly increase."
— — — **Eiji Morishita, Founder of Speak Your Genius**

THE DIAMOND HEALING METHOD: GET HEALTHY NO MATTER WHAT YOUR DOCTOR SAYS

Dr. Anastasia Chopelas

Dedication

This book is dedicated to my wonderful
parents, Alec and Zafiria* Chopelas.
It was their encouragement and enthusiasm
that inspired me to take this path.

Gratitude and Acknowledgments:
My husband, Noel Shelton, and
my daughter, Marika Blue,
have been ongoing supports
through the process of writing this book.

Table of Contents

Disclaimer

The information in this book is to be used for educational purposes only. This book is not intended to replace the expert advice of your own personal physician or another licensed health care practitioner.

Before taking any supplement or starting any exercise program, consult your physician. Your physician is your partner to helping you achieve good health. A good physician is worth his/her weight in gold.

There are several complimentary bonus materials mentioned throughout the book that will help you on your healing journey. Sign up at http://scientifichealer.com/book-bonus/

This includes:
Chapter bonus: 18 tips for staying fit and healthy while on the road. Plus four other bonuses including free audio, food tracker, etc.

This book may not be altered, given away or freely copied without express permission.

Foreword by Robert Allen

*"Most of the time our stress is useless. It's because we don't
see the outcome of things. God does."*
Amanda Penland

It is my pleasure to introduce this ground-breaking book connecting energy medicine to science. This connection shows that your health and quality of life are clearly dependent on your behavior and interactions.

When I met Anastasia, she was fresh from retiring a forty-year career as a physics professor and researcher, where she studied the vibrations and energetics of matter. I was intrigued to discover that she was now a full-time energy healer and had developed a method all her own that incorporates much of her research topic into understanding human health on all levels.

You may be surprised to learn that all the things that we call spiritual healing have a basis in science- something that's measurable and reproducible.

Anastasia joined my Fortune in You program because she had been healing in a private practice with incredible success, making medical miracles an every day occurrence. Her determination to help as many people as possible meant that she needed to learn how to most effectively spread her message. She has worked diligently learning and participating in this program.

I have watched Anastasia transform from a lecturer at a podium to someone who connects with the people in the room and moves them to actions. She does all this because she cares deeply about transforming the health of the planet.

She is rightly the "Scientific Healer," because very few others practicing energy medicine understand what is occurring at the atomic level. Her clients have experienced profound changes in their lives, with over 250 medical miracles and transformations. Some have been pulled back from the brink of death and others have had their quality of life dramatically improved. Many of these stories you'll read in this book.

The exciting aspect of her work is that she has systematized it with the skills she learned as a scientist and teacher so anyone can learn it. Many of the practices are simple and easy to incorporate into your life.

In this introductory book, Anastasia describes the Diamond Method in practical terms, showing you how your stress depends on seven different factors. The stress has a direct correlation to your energy and ultimately your health and wellbeing. Major studies have shown that major stresses are directly correlated to major illnesses.

You'll learn that you come with an energetic blueprint for perfect health and that it is the influences from the seven factors that cause the deviations from good health. She calls this your programming. So many of you believe that you are stuck with your programming but with good energetic practices, you can reprogram yourself to better health, better relationships, better careers and even more wealth.

Anastasia's family of origin inspired this work. At first, it became about healing herself from major illness. Then she was able to help her family members -- many of whom had struggled with major health crises and "incurable" illnesses. Lives were brought to a standstill. Her family focused on their illnesses instead of enjoying each other. The revolutionary Diamond Healing Method is the result of her research. She fervently wishes this work helps families come together and so they can be healthy families again.

Robert G. Allen,
Corona Del Mar, CA
January, 2015

Introduction

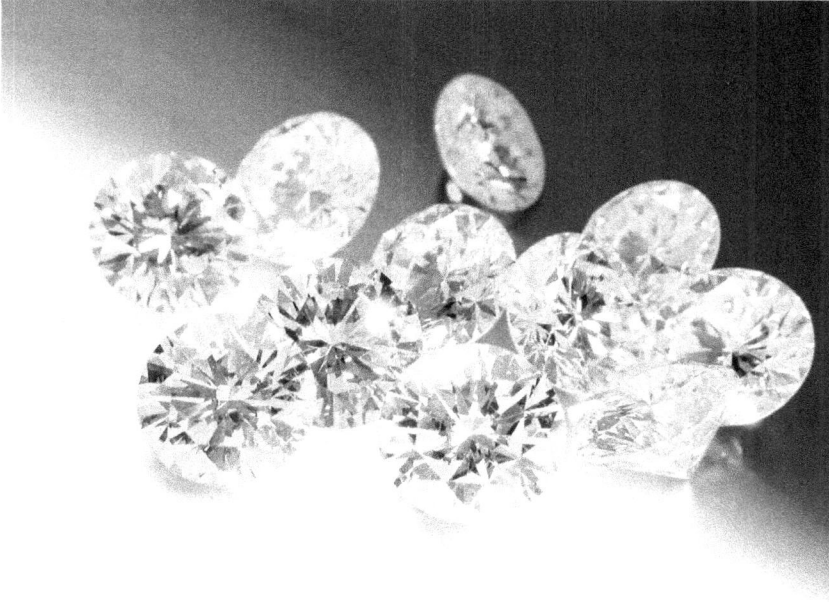

"I have lived a long life and had many troubles . . . most of which never happened."
Mark Twain

What is this book about?

I woke up one day over 20 years ago to the realization that despite my best efforts, I was a sick person. I had no energy with up to two good hours a day, I had trouble keeping my weight in check, high blood pressure, a lot of body pain, I had a huge abdominal tumor, and I was constantly getting ill. During the previous six-month period, I was sick in bed more than I was up and about. While this might be something that a person who had abused their body might suffer, I had eaten healthy, run 6 miles before breakfast every day for years, and should have been by all accounts, super healthy.

I was a single mom with two children ages 6 and 9, and in addition to their needs, I had a big house to take care of. I lived in Germany, where my German wasn't fluent enough to carry on adult conversations. I had a full-blown career as a research scientist, which meant long hours and hard work. I had an almost ex-husband that wasn't making things easy.

The question I kept asking myself: How did I get there and how was I going to get out of it?

That day was the day I started on a journey of discovery. It was in my nature to research everything down to the last detail, so I started with discovering the cause of my large tumor and what I could do to shrink it. As I learned by reading medical textbooks, research papers, and books on "natural" health and healing, there wasn't much known about it. I even went online and talked to other women with the same issue. I sent out a survey to them to discover a unifying cause for the problem. I had hundreds of results to pore over: I read thousands of pages of surveys and books. I found that there wasn't one unifying dietary, body weight (fat versus lean), exercise or not, water drinker or not, alcohol use/abuse or not, no one could put their finger on a particular cause. The medical community said they were spontaneous and no cause known. Being a scientist, I knew there had to be a cause, because we are wired to heal and not be ill. I knew the cause was just not clear yet.

To get to the punch line before this story gets too long, it turns out that each one of these women in my survey were experiencing stress in some form or other. Many of them had low self-esteem, were trying to prove they were worthy, and were abusive to themselves and their bodies. They also put up with abusive partners, petty tyrant bosses, or had other toxic relationships. I could see clearly that their nerves were stretched taut with stress with all the chaos and strife in their lives.

I realized that I too was a poster child for stress as I was trying to be superwoman and living a life with clenched teeth for the verbal abuse I had allowed in my life, the amount of responsibility I felt for everything and the daily grind that had become my life. I felt trapped and nothing I did was ever good enough for myself and the others around me: this was a message that followed me from childhood.

Now, twenty plus years later, this path of discovery has led me to some pretty profound truths and a place where I feel I can live authentically, without clenched teeth, truly enjoying every day of my life. Now in my 60s, I am pain free, medication free, energetic, strong and able to do things I couldn't even do in my 20s. In this journey, I have found that stress manifests itself due to seven causes (it's really three, but seven separate issues) that if they are resolved, profound changes take place in your life. This book is a result of my 20-year journey of discovery.

This discovery includes that the vast majority of illness and disease comes from stress. The stress means you are out of alignment with your perfect energetic blueprint for health you came into the world with. So, let's look at some stress facts and come back around to this point. The Diamond Healing Method addresses all seven factors that cause stress.

Stress facts

It is estimated that up to 2/3 of the adults in the United States have overworked adrenal glands due to stressful lives. This is staggering. This statistic means you are probably one of them. Fortunately, there are solutions that you can fit into your busy day that will help reduce the stress and get you functioning well again.

Here is why you should worry about it: Stress causes major illnesses. It's actually worse than that; it also destroys relationships and careers.

During my worst stress, I heard all the messages. Manage stress, reduce stress, de-stress. Meditate, take it easy, stop to smell the flowers, etc. I would ask myself, what does that all mean? How do I fit one more thing into my crazy schedule? I know I didn't have a clue even though I was living my life with clenched teeth. I didn't even know what it meant to be relaxed, I had lived stressed for so long

For those of you who are stressed, the very idea of taking on one more project, fitting one more thing into your day or changing your habits from the ones you are accustomed to is just, well, more stress.

This book is a new approach to stress. You see, stress is additive. But so are the solutions you can do in small steps.

It isn't just your mind-set; it is also your environment and your interaction with it, whether it's other people, your surroundings or what you put in your body. It's also about how you treat yourself and what you tell yourself every day. When you look at it this way, it's really all about energy management, which is what this book describes. Small adjustments in your day, your interactions with your environment, others, or yourself can add up to big positive effects on your internal stress levels. Here, you'll learn small simple adjustment techniques that add up to major improvements in your life.

What are some of the signs that you are stressed? Can you identify with any of these?

  ! You wake up tired even after eight hours of sleep.
  ! You are overwhelmed trying to fit so much into your life that the thought of taking on one more task sends you into a downward spiral of stress.
  ! You're short tempered and impatient with so many people and activities during your day.
  ! You've forgotten how to laugh, joke or kid around with your friends and family.
  ! You crave sweet or salty foods.
  ! You feel you can't afford to take a day off, that all your activities and the people around you are more important than you are.
  ! You've gained a lot (or lost a lot) of weight because you were eating without paying attention to what you were eating OR you forgot to eat.
  ! You seem to suffer from colds and the sniffles way too often or have a lot of body pain such as lower back or joint pain. It's chronic and the doctor can't seem to find any physical cause. You don't recover easily.
  ! You have a major illness or high blood pressure, high cholesterol and other "middle age" conditions.
  ! You suffer a lot of headaches.
  ! Things that didn't used to bother you drive you crazy now.

! You are sensitive to sounds, especially if there are two or three of them, like the radio, conversation and background sounds.
! You can't figure out why you've hit a roadblock in your life. After all, you're working hard to get ahead.
! Your current behavior is causing your relationships to deteriorate.
! You might even be considering dangerous activities such as illegal drugs, risky behavior, or affairs just to feel alive again.

If you said yes to any of these, you could use some relief: please keep reading to discover how.

The cost of stress:

Now that you've seen what an over-stressed life looks like, here are some of the consequences of not taking care of it. While stressed, you are caught in a vicious cycle that can cause serious, lasting damage to your health.

Unresolved stress, the kind you haven't dealt with and eliminated from your body and mind, is sometimes called *chronic* or *toxic stress*. This sustained stress overrides your body's natural abilities to bounce back. This activates the adrenal glands that pump out stress hormones, and keeps them at high levels. In this, the so-called sympathetic state of your nervous system, **your body is using its resources**. As this state continues, your immune system is suppressed to the point that it leaves you unable to heal well and you become vulnerable to colds, flu, and a much worse set of illnesses and conditions.

As toxic stress continues, your body's ability to produce cortisol and another adrenal hormone, DHEA (dehydroepiandrosterone), becomes diminished. You become even less able to respond in an appropriate way to stressors and become unable to end the stress cycle.

Here are some of the prices you pay for toxic stress in the short term:

o Suppressed immune system, increasing risk of infections

- Reduced ability of the body to repair itself
- Slower metabolism – inhibition of thyroid hormones
- Reduced ability to absorb vital nutrients

You may experience the following physical symptoms:
- Recurring headaches
- Vague aches and pains
- Dizziness
- Heartburn
- Muscle tension
- Dry mouth
- Excessive perspiration
- Pounding heart
- Insomnia
- Fatigue

The long-term price you pay is even heavier:
- Acceleration of the aging process with a shortened lifespan
- Weight gain
- Increased risk of digestive problems (ulcers, colitis), osteoporosis, high blood pressure, high cholesterol, heart disease, and even cancer. In other words, you experience a much lower quality of life.
- Difficulties in relationships and big losses in future earnings

In this condition, your brain runs out of the feel-good brain chemicals, you experience the following:
- Anxiety, fear, restlessness
- Irritability, anger
- Depression
- Insecurity
- Loss of sex drive
- Excessive eating, smoking, drinking, or drug use

This book is for you if:
- ✓ You are already making some changes in your life to improve it.

✔ You are willing to make further changes to get your life, your joy, and your energy back.

✔ You are creative, imaginative, and are willing to look for solutions that don't fit inside the box of conventional medicine as long as they work and are safe to use.

✔ You want to ensure your future health and well being by spending up to half an hour a day doing simple mental and physical exercises to gain more hours of clarity and energy.

✔ Your doctor has told you there is nothing more he/she has to offer you but you can hardly believe that.

This book is not for you if:

x You are not willing to make simple changes in your life that will help you move forward.

x You are not open to new ideas on how to improve your health, relationships and career.

x You think your life is fine the way it is, even though your spouse can't stand you, your kids don't want to be around you and your coworkers avoid you.

x You are convinced that conventional (Western) medicine has the only options available to improving your health and well-being.

x You are not already trying new things to help you get out of the rut you are in.

If you find this book is for you, there is no time like *now* to get started. You'll discover in the pages of this book that illness starts long before you see the symptoms. Isn't *now* a good time to get started learning to stay healthy, vibrant and productive way into the future?

What is stress anyway?

Most people are not aware that stress has a very specific scientific definition. It is pressure or tension exerted on an object. If you think about it, this is a much broader definition than "a state of emotional or mental strain due to demanding circumstances," found in many dictionaries or to put it another way, disappointing yourself or others.

Biologically, the definition of stress is the body's method of reacting to a challenge, which is very similar to the physics definition. It specifically results in a fight or flight response, which means sympathetic nervous system activation. It increases breathing and heart rate, elevates blood pressure, and raises blood-sugar levels, preparing the body for either self-defense or escape.

This broadens the definition of stress when it comes to wellness and illness. Why? Because anything that sends the body into that fight-or-flight state activates the sympathetic nervous system. That means your adrenal glands are pouring out their hormones and your body is using its resources instead of replenishing them. It's not just all in your head; it's all parts of your being.

There's another important mechanism that takes place when you are chronically stressed: your blood sugar levels rise and then abruptly fall. That's because adrenaline and cortisol dump sugar into your bloodstream, and in an hour or two your blood sugar crashes. This is a serious problem because 20% of your body's entire intake of glucose fuels your brain, so when your sugars crash, you start feeling foggy, nervous, tired, and irritable. Good decision-making becomes difficult. Wildly fluctuating blood sugar also causes other serious health issues such as high cholesterol and inflammation, weight gain and the problems associated with it.

Because of this, your long-term exposure to stress can lead to serious health problems and your ability to even think clearly is compromised. Chronic stress disrupts nearly every system in your body. It can raise your blood pressure, suppress the immune system, increase your risk of heart attack and stroke, contribute to infertility, and speed up the aging process. Long-term stress can even rewire your brain, leaving you more vulnerable to anxiety and depression.

If your body is using your resources more than it is restoring or replenishing them, illness and disease result.

Prior to illness and disease showing up, physical changes will manifest themselves, sometimes years before. We can measure the changes in your body using simple devices that measure the field of the body. The results of these stress induced changes are often obvious: overwhelm, fatigue, burnout, frequent colds, muscle cramps, headaches, depression, and pain. These are all due to stress. If you let the stress go on for a long period of time, it leads to chronic conditions, such as heart disease and cancer, the two largest causes of death in the United States.

There are many more circumstances in your life that set the stress response in motion than are generally recognized. In this book, using the Diamond Method program, we identify the seven most common stress factors. It isn't just about slowing down and smelling the roses, though that helps. It isn't just about getting enough rest, though that helps. It isn't just about solving your relationship difficulties, though that helps too. We'll address all seven stress factors and work to quickly resolve them without years of therapy or dangerous medical treatments.

There are a host of side benefits that come along with getting our bodies from the sympathetic or stressed state into the parasympathetic or rejuvenating state. These side effects are typical amongst my private clients:

- ✓ You'll notice that your sleep will be productive and you'll feel rested in the morning, fully energized and ready to roll.
- ✓ You'll notice all your relationships improve, including your coworkers, bosses and subordinates as well as those in your personal life.
- ✓ If you are a boss, your business will run more smoothly.
- ✓ You might even find the love of your life whether or not you are looking for them.
- ✓ Or your current relationships all improve.
- ✓ Your business and personal phone will ring off the hook.

Decisions will be easier because your mind will be clearer. Your mind won't be clouded by all the "white noise" around that stress causes. You might even notice your financial situation improving, with income rising because people are magnetized to you. They want to work with you, winning big contracts you thought might be out of reach, or you might be promoted because your bosses see value in what you offer.

You'll even notice that a lot of the little aches and pains in your body go away or chronic conditions that you thought you were destined to live with seem to improve and even fully resolve, such as high blood pressure or arthritis or worse.

Sound too good to be true?

Bear with me as I show you how stress, not just emotional stress, but physical stress on the body, once alleviated, will allow you to reach your highest potential. It doesn't take years of talk therapy or some magic pill or formula or hours of your time. The methods here are rapid. We use a proven transformational protocol called the Diamond Method, developed over years of research.

There are seven ways in which the stress response is set up in the body. By addressing these factors, one at a time, your future course is altered. Hundreds of my private clients can attest to this.

I'm sure you've heard the expression: think outside the box. I believe we need to throw away the box and start all over again. We require new innovative approaches to solving our problems especially after they've arrived because conventional methods have not fulfilled the promise of finding solutions.

After years of talk therapy, medications, surgeries, etc., many people are barely further along than when they started and are usually much poorer financially as a result. Some of my clients told me they lost their homes seeking conventional and traditional treatments. The number one reason people file for bankruptcy in this country is insurmountable medical debt. And to make matters worse, the medical treatments and the bills incurred are just as stressful as the physical causes if not more. Indeed, the third most common reason for mortality in the United States after heart disease and cancer is medical and prescription error. I don't believe we should throw out the baby with the bathwater, but consider a prudent balance between the two.

So, what is the solution? Consider the somewhat gloomy prospect offered by conventional medicine alone and how insurance covers the cost of these despite their not being effective. The medical establishment is counting on us to buy into this system and it disparages other concepts of health and wellbeing. If you step back and look at the situation from a high altitude, you will discover that you have the power to change it after all and you can change it without spending thousands of dollars for many years to come. At this high altitude, you can see that the three important factors in our health crises in the United States, the exorbitant cost, the lack of effectiveness and or medical error, and poor quality of life while on it, can be changed by simple changes in our daily habits, our thinking and our interactions with our environment.

How transformation can occur

There are two important discoveries that took place about a hundred years ago that revealed the basis of stress in the body, that of Einstein and that of Burr. To understand how these impact us, first, remember that stress is your body's reaction to a challenge, which simultaneously alters your physical, chemical, mental and emotional states. To challenge the body, you would apply an energy to it, an energy counter to its natural flow.

Your body then works very hard to hold things in stasis, which is another way of saying that it is trying to maintain the status quo, to bring things back into balance again. If you look at a challenge this way, the definition of stress can also include abusing your body with toxic food or drink, lack of sleep, a non-nurturing environment, including toxic people, toxic air, water, and behaving in a way that's against your own inner compass.

Energy is applied to you to create the stress, your body expends energy to counteract it.

What is energy exactly?

In any physics textbook, energy is defined as the ability to do work: this means you can transform something from one thing to another. Every rock, mineral, chair, piece of metal, couch, or any other inanimate object contains characteristic energies because their atoms are vibrating even if you can't see them moving. We know this by measurements made in the laboratory on any material. The frequencies of their vibration depend on their composition, bonding and temperature. One of the ways that energy of this innate vibration shows up is as a field around the object.

For living entities, plant or animal including you, the energy fields are even larger due to the trillions of reactions that go on in each of your 38 trillion cells every single day. Now that we know that there are energy fields around all objects, let's look at even a bigger picture of energy.

Energy is all there is.

Matter is mostly empty space. If we condensed the entire Earth down to its component nucleons (protons and neutrons), it would just be a (very heavy) 75 yards across. Condense it further to the density of a black hole, it would occupy just a fraction of an inch. The Earth is the size it is because its contained energy keeps it expanded. Your mind cannot even comprehend how much energy that is.

Furthermore, the component particles of atoms, what we could consider as "matter" can even be defined as energy. This is the first of the important discoveries: Einstein discovered through his observation of radioactive decay that all matter is basically energy. It is expressed in his famous equation: $E = mc^2$, where E is energy, m is mass and c is the speed of light (which is a constant and never varies). This equation is basically saying that matter is energy.

If matter is energy, then it should behave as other energy does. There needs to be a way to measure the energy of matter, not only with their mass and velocity, which is difficult when they're that small and fast.

Shortly after another of Einstein's discovery: that light behaves as particles, French scientist Louis de Broglie hypothesized that since light can behave as if it were matter, solid matter may also have the properties of light. This means it has frequencies/wavelengths that should be dependent on its energy of movement, in other words, its mass and velocity.

Experiments at the quantum/atomic level proved this concept in which the components of atoms: electrons, protons and neutrons demonstrated wave properties according to de Broglie's ideas. Indeed, wavelengths of these particles were measured when they were subjected to the same experiments as light, such as diffraction experiments. They were excited and intrigued to be able to measure the wavelength of matter.

These outrageous results put the whole world of physics on its ear. Imagine that a baseball being pitched to a batter has a wavelength and it vibrates at a frequency. That means that everything has a frequency. It was out of these revolutionary ideas (and others) that quantum physics was grounded.

Despite what you may think you know about how things work, there is a world of connection and energy that you probably hadn't considered existed. Even physicists that have studied these phenomena for decades are unable to explain them fully; they can only describe what they observe and they may even find equations that describe their observations. There is no one yet that fully understands wave-particle duality, gravity or light.

It is with this in mind that you begin to see that there is more than meets the eye with regard to how anything works on an energetic level. As mentioned above, the experimental evidence for subtle energies and fields around objects has been around for nearly a century. Now, you'll be able to put this idea in the context of stress on the body with the next set of discoveries.

Do humans have measurable fields?

At about the same time Einstein and de Broglie were making their observations, Dr. H.S. Burr was measuring the energy fields around living tissue. He found that even around an embryo, the size of the field was as large as it would be as an adult and it is symmetric about the brain and spinal cord. The field is essentially an energetic blueprint that the organism grows into. That seemed to defy the laws of physics. It would be expected that the field would grow with the organism, not be the same size as the adult to begin with.

If you pose the question another way, how does the body know which way to grow? How does it know what size it is to be? Obviously this information is contained somewhere in your body. It is imprinted onto your being and is measurable by simple devices.

Dr. Burr made some other discoveries that were equally as intriguing. In one experiment, he infected mice with cancer cells and noted that their energy fields changed (they shrank) within 24 hours but the cancer didn't manifest until much later. This means the energy inside the body shifts as illness takes hold, the field shrinks as the energy depletes.

It is not always a foregone conclusion that the disease will actually manifest. As we've seen over and over again in studies: if people are exposed to the same virus or germ, each person reacts differently to it. What is it that those who stayed healthy have that the ones that become ill and die don't?

In short, it is your resilience from stress. The question is: how exactly can you improve that? Your resilience is how you and your body manage the challenges and how you dissipate the stress it creates. Since stress directly affects your energy fields, it also stands to reason that anything improving your energy fields could dissipate the stress on your body, bringing it back to its original calm state. There are three major steps to managing your stress using simple, straightforward techniques that anyone can do in just minutes a day.

What is the Diamond Method?

The Diamond Method is a fresh upgrade to energy medicine that incorporates modern scientific knowledge including filters, mathematical functions, quantum physics, biochemistry, and modern discoveries of nutrition into ancient healing techniques.

Application of these protocols in my private practice has allowed 250 people to be healed and to produce what other people would call medical miracles. But even more astonishing than the medical miracles are the personal transformations that include dramatic increases in abundance, not only in health, but wealth and relationships. In other words, you'll see massive changes in "love and money", where incomes have increased by up to factors of six and single men and women have met the loves of their lives. Bringing all of your physical, emotional, and spiritual energies from discord to their full potential means your stress levels go way down and you become who you were always meant to be, healthy, happy and abundant.

In my work with hundreds of people, I have observed that illness, unhappiness, loneliness, poor marriages, poor work performance and even poverty can be traced to one form of stress or another. Rather than get involved in esoteric concepts that few understand and accept, what is really happening in the body is that the adrenal glands are constantly firing and being over stimulated, causing the energy producing systems in the body (the mitochondria, the liver, and the digestive system) to become overtaxed then depleted. This is reflected as a measurable drop in the energy field of the body. The physical body then takes its time to transform to the new "ill" energy pattern.

While this is not a step by step follow the numbers instruction book for how to heal something specific, it gives you insights and instructions on many aspects of energy medicine. Each one of the chapters taken alone can improve your life. There is a summary of the protocol I use to get people started on a healing journey in Appendix II.

You may have already heard of the topics I mention and discuss. If you have, let them serve as a reminder. Remember, we all get this information from the same source, it is downloaded from the Divine. Otherwise, why would the information from so many healers and sources be so similar? We can all tap into it.

The only thing you have to keep in mind is that intent is everything. Intend the energy to flow, it does. Intend to direct the energy to go in a place, it does. Intend to get better, you will. You do have to take steps to change your life, that's the action on your part.

The solution is simple but not easy.

Our interaction with the environment is complex because we do it on so many levels. We interact physically with food, rest, water, and our environment. We react emotionally to everything we see, from people to situations even our likes and dislikes such as what color to paint a room or what we like to wear. And we react spiritually via our moral compass, the sublime energies that we are bombarded with, even though most of us unaware of their existence. Untangling this web comes down to understanding how we interact with our environment, others, and ourselves on every level.

Reading on H.S. Burr in Wikipedia (http://en.wikipedia.org/wiki/ Harold_Saxton_Burr)

1. You have the ability to change your future

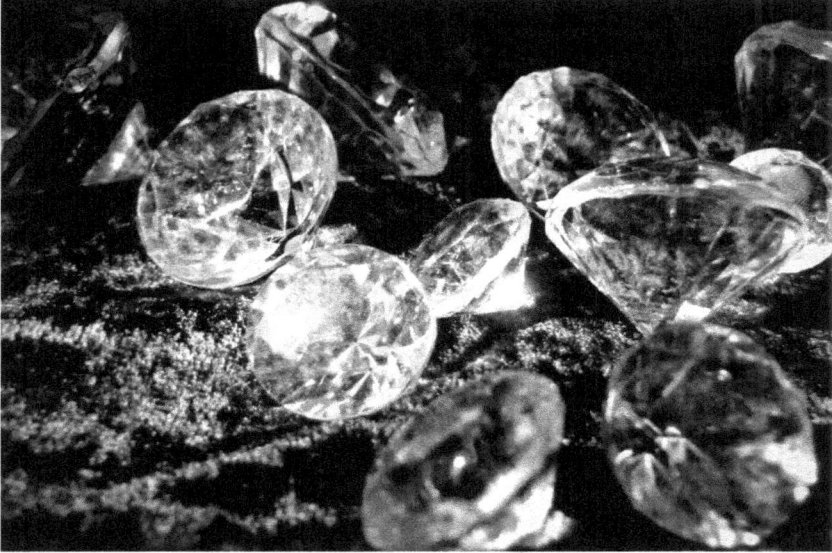

"Please don't tell me to relax
it's only my tension that's holding me together."
Jane Seabrook, *Furry Logic Wild Wisdom*

You have the power to create the life you want. You'll find that your thoughts and intentions allow you to manifest great things with them. You'll discover the importance of your emotions to your physical health, your connection to other people, and your ability to lead and engage others in your visions. You'll also learn how you can process out negative emotions quickly and easily and protect yourself from the negativity of others. You'll find **you** can create a healthy, vibrant and abundant life despite what you may have been told or have read somewhere.

The biggest stumbling block that most of us have is that we don't believe it fully. Your self-doubts and fears and sometimes the doubts and fears of others are holding you back. We get in our own way. That is the root of emotional stress. It doesn't matter which aspect of your life you want to move forward. It all creates stress in your body.

For example, despite Bill's good health, career training, and intermittent financial success, when he came to me, his life was in turmoil and his language about himself was full of doubt as to whether he'd be successful or not. His stress levels made it nearly impossible to see how he could solve his dilemmas in a short amount of time so he could pursue his real dream, teaching others how to help themselves become financially independent as he had.

Bill divorced a few years back and was in the throes of another split, this time from Suzanne, a one-year relationship that he wanted to continue on some level. Suzanne had decided to move across the country and was hoping that Bill would follow. Bill's dilemma was he would be leaving his nearly grown children, a business and properties on one coast to relocate to another.

Each coast called to him and he felt torn: just this decision alone occupied much of his thoughts. He also wanted to sell his current business while helping his several employees keep their incomes. He wasn't sure which properties to liquidate, had no idea which city to settle in, and did not know whether he should stay in the relationship with Suzanne, as he found her to be a lovely woman and admired her values. He also felt he couldn't desert her because she was a very needy woman. The stress in Bill's life was tremendous, as fear and doubt affected every area of his life. He thought it would take months to resolve everything.

Bill came to me at this crossroads as a private client for spiritual guidance and clarity in his life. Through the work we did together, which included relationship clearings and releasing emotional blocks, he realized how much he was living his life according to outer voices: he felt led around, he spent a lot of time worried and he saw no clear or quick solutions. In his relationship, he realized there lacked enough mutual agreement and compromise for major life-altering decisions such as moving 3000 miles away.

In one month's time, he managed to resolve selling his business without hurting his current employees, he received good offers on the properties he needed to sell, was able to leave his relationship with Suzanne behind amicably, and decided where to live. He elected to stay on the same coast as his children, started a new teaching/coaching business that is taking off, and he connected confidently with other successful coaches because his program perfectly supplements theirs and is now developing programs with them. He is moving forward with ease and confidence instead of doubt and worry.

The level of stress that Bill was feeling is now replaced with an exhilaration and excitement as he looks forward to realizing his dreams rather than being stuck in the past. The quick resolution allows him to move forward to help others realize their dreams on a much bigger scale than ever before. And last, Bill is finally realizing that he can find a partner that isn't so needy. Instead he is looking forward to finding someone mutually supportive when the time is right.

What this book is really about

Here, you'll discover the principles that Bill learned that allowed him to move quickly out of the stress of several unresolved and dissatisfying issues. This includes understanding the basic energetic building blocks of your being and how to take care of them, an essential element to taming your stress. This last year, amongst my private clients and students, I have helped co-create over 250 medical miracles by helping them manage their stress levels and personal energy. It released them from the bondages of their past, including belief systems, self-sabotage, and emotional blocks. It also helped their organs, glands and systems heal. As a side effect, both their personal lives and professional lives have changed for the better. It has helped them propel their lives forward in directions that they hadn't thought possible, or only dreamed of.

You'll find that once health returns by managing your environment and personal stress, seemingly magical things happen with your life. Ingrid, a TV producer, was living a very stressful life with an ailing parent at home, running a bar/restaurant to make some income to keep her afloat between jobs. She was feeling overworked and exhausted.

She was proposing several show ideas to investors in this state and, as you might have guessed, most of them didn't succeed. She had only closed one show deal in the six months prior to working with me. After two months with me, she felt much more comfortable in her situation, her physical energy improved and she closed six show deals in that time. This proceeded by healing the energy systems of her body and clearing old emotional and relationship patterns. Essentially, she changed her income by a factor of six.

You'll see that it's fully in your hands whether you stay stuck or move forward.

You may at this point be wondering exactly how I went from a very technical science to a healing art. You'll find I haven't really left science and I prefer to think of what I do as scientific healing.

How it all began

I'm most often asked, "how can you, a successful physicist, have gone from a "hard-core" science based in facts to something that seems to be almost at the opposite end of the spectrum?" In reality, it seems as if my life was guided to do this work because of all the things I learned along the way. This process began at an early age. When I was seven years old, I received two gifts that changed the course of my life.

The first gift opened my mind to infinite possibilities: My dad brought home a map of the universe showing the planets, moons, sun, and asteroids and hung it on the kitchen wall. I was so totally awestruck to see that instead of being this enormous place, Earth was just a tiny speck in this vast and seemingly infinite universe. My curiosity was roused. Wow, I thought, there are other planets! They're so big, so unusual, made out of other things, not rocks but ice and gas. How could that be? They had a lot of moons, no moons or rings, unlike Earth. Even tiny Mars had two moons.

My imagination was set free.

As time went on, I found that we are not just limited by what we can observe nearby, there is a whole other universe waiting to be explored. We can easily see some objects, but others are only observable by the effects they create or the filter/lens we observe them with. An example of this is a black hole. It is a massive object, which has gravitational pull is so strong, that light cannot escape it. Hence, it is black. We can't see it but the tremendous gravity effects are obvious if you look for them.

I stared at that map, shown above, by the hour, memorizing every fact, image, and concept on it. I wanted to know so much more. I decided then that I was going to study science. And indeed, years later, I got my PhD in physical chemistry, then spent decades studying the universe, reporting my findings at scientific conferences and publishing in scholarly articles and book chapters.

In fact, in that study of the universe, I studied the energetics of matter, the vibrations of minerals and other materials, quantum mechanics and thermodynamics. I studied the universe from microscopic to macroscopic, understanding atoms and molecules on the most detailed level and how they affected matter at larger scales. I probed samples with lasers after compressing them between two diamonds. I teased the information out of small crystals and interpreted the data and applied it to model the Earth and other planets. I am well respected for the work I published and considered one of the top experts in the energetics of matter under extreme conditions.

The long hours in the lab and on research prepared me well for understanding human energetics and has allowed me to explore it in ways that were unprejudiced by "conventional wisdom". The methods in this book are much like the experiments in the laboratory: probe, experiment, and result. If the result is something other than what was wanted after trying something, alter the protocol until your desired result is achieved. As with the universe and its exploration, each discovery is mind boggling, such as the discovery of enormous terrestrial planets revolving around giant suns at a breakneck pace. These could not be imagined until the (very recent) discovery of 1900+ exo-planets, that is, planets revolving around distant star systems. This number grows exponentially every year.

The second gift

The second gift that changed my life was a book on the human body I received for Christmas after my seventh birthday: it was a thick volume on all the systems, glands and organs and their functions (see below). I loved that book: I still have it. I read through it hundreds of times, also memorizing every picture, every word, and

28

every idea in it. I was also fascinated by how many things were tucked into the body, how all the parts fit neatly and how everything functioned separately and as a whole. By the time I was eight, I knew every system in the body and what it did. This began a lifelong fascination on health, fitness, and discovering how the body can best function.

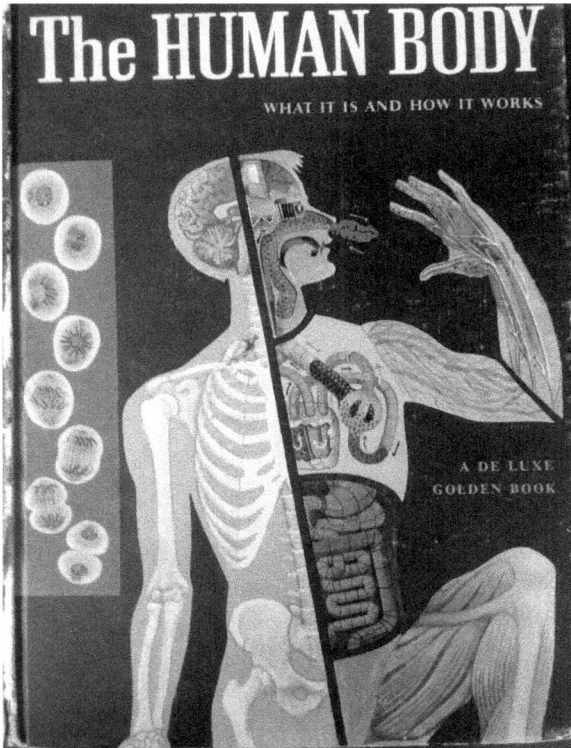

Shortly after this, when my dad discovered he had thalassemia, an inherited anemia found in people native to the Adriatic Sea region, he went about searching for answers to feeling better. In an era (ca. 1960) when Wonder Bread and Corn Flakes were the normal diet, we were eating homemade multigrain bread and whole grain hot cereals. At that time, there was no such thing as Yoplait, frozen yoghurt, or yoghurt chocolate, and no one even heard of yoghurt. Yet we were eating unflavored, un-sugared homemade yoghurt daily. Wholesome fruits and vegetables, often homegrown, fresh protein sources (not lunch meats), and nuts/seeds were daily staples.

So, in addition to studying the body, I also learned about nutrition, supplements, exercise, and rest at a very early age.

This fascination with the body and health continued throughout my life. I developed good health habits early. Of all my friends in college, I was the only one that didn't eat pizza, hamburgers, and drink sugared sodas. I would go to parties and be the only one that didn't eat all the goodies. From high school on, I ran 6 miles before breakfast, ate very well and stayed at 120 lbs., which on a 65" tall body is lean and healthy.

I was full of energy, enthusiasm, and loved everything about my life. I was doing my dream job as a research scientist, lived in awesome locations like Germany, got to travel everywhere to speak to scientists all over the world. I got to learn fluent German, practice my French and Spanish. I went to Australia, Japan, all through Europe and the US, Canada, and Mexico.

During my time as a research scientist, I studied the vibrations and energetics of minerals at high pressures and temperatures. It allowed me to probe how the universe was formed, how we came into existence, and what planets and stars and everything in between are made of. Believe it or not, the scientific principles I learned then now help to solve health issues at the causal level. As you saw in the introduction, I also had to live through health crises myself and necessity is the real reason for my move from science to scientific healing.

The story behind the story

My health crash over 20 years ago left me depressed. I wanted again to be as active and vibrant as I had in the first 41 years of my life. Given that my parents taught me extraordinary lessons about healthy eating and exercise, I had indeed expected to be well for a lot longer than I was. Over the next ten to 15 years, I was afflicted with the following: high blood pressure, high cholesterol, fibroid tumor, severe inflammatory arthritis, migraines, and a weariness that made me wonder how I was going to survive.

With my health in trouble, I also didn't seem to ever get back on my feet financially despite my working hard, being highly educated, talented, and succeeding in some ways but not being able to go through life with the grace and ease I had hoped for.

I had to take a good look at my life and prioritize my activities and figure out how I was going to win my health back while in this fragile state.

As any good researcher would, I spent a great deal of time working at understanding allergies, fibroid tumors, blood pressure, cholesterol, arthritis, lack of energy, thyroid, blood sugar control, weight control, psychology and relationships, addictions, stress management, homeopathy, naturopathy and energy medicine. Slowly, taking care of each problem one by one, I was able to bring my health back into line.

It took years to wade through research reports, skewed results, skewed reports, and separate the mythology from the facts. It wasn't easy because so many things that are accepted as healthy are in actuality harmful.

Each step I took, I had a big internal resistance to it because my life was stretched to the limits already. But each time I succeeded (and I did not succeed 100% of the time), my health improved. I worked hard at it because I wanted to have the energy to be a good mother to my two young children, to see them grow up and have them avoid the same kind of health crisis as they aged.

In examining these factors one by one, I discovered there was an overarching factor that impacted my wellbeing and health: stress. For example, the big discovery that even eating the foods we are mildly allergic to will cause our adrenal glands to fire meant that our stress levels will rise with issues that have nothing to do with emotional fortitude and expectations. In examining other factors that could lead to stress, it turns out that nearly everything that doesn't agree with your being evokes stress. In summary, seven interactions that we have with the outside world or ourselves contribute to our health, well-being, relationships and success in our careers. These are addressed in this book.

The transition from scientist to scientific healer

During this period of searching while ill, I discovered alternative medicine. I was lucky because I lived in Germany through much of this time, where homeopathy and naturopathy are much more developed and respected than in the US. It was through some pretty miraculous results on my own problems that I began to take these seriously.

I also discovered how to feel human energy fields, as well as, how to alter my field and that of others. Remember, Dr. Burr discovered using a simple instrument, that your energy field changes long before illness begins. You can see this for yourself by looking at the difference between someone that is vitally alive to those that are stressed out or even ill. In the one case, their eyes are vibrantly alive and smiling even when they're quiet, their skin glows and they walk around strong and confidently while in the other case, their eyes are dull and even bored, their skin dull with no color and the gait is slow and painful looking.

You can feel the edge of their fields (or measure them with an instrument). The former's field would be strong, large and complete while the latter's would be close to the body and even non-existent in some places. This matches with Dr. H.S. Burr's observations.

What you are about to learn in this book is that you have the ability to alter your field around your body in such a way to help bring health, vitality, clarity, and calmness back to yourself. Just as the field reacts to the body's condition, the body reacts to the field's condition. By improving the energy of the field, the body slowly comes back to a healthy state. There are so many ways to do this: seven to be exact.

Ways to improve your field that you've already heard about include improving diet, exercising, better sleep habits, and improving what we put on our body. As I learned via reading and studying with teachers, I learned that there were other ways to strengthen the body field. You can also use intent, prayer, gratitude, imagery, and drawing in energy from the environment (such as from the sun) as long as you are open to it. I found I could help others work with their own fields and helped them facilitate it. There have been a number of serious academic and medical studies showing that intent, mood, gratitude, prayer, and good relationships contribute to your well-being. It basically amounts to reducing your stress reaction to a given situation.

Some of the miracles that I mentioned earlier started happening almost immediately after applying these principles. It seemed so obvious after knowing exactly how the body is put together from my study of physiology, biochemistry, and anatomy as well as a clear understanding of the energy structures of the body.

These miracles included correcting hemochromatosis (excess blood iron levels) very quickly, calming ADHD down, improving autism dramatically, improving pain from fibromyalgia, eliminating severe gastritis in minutes, relaxing stubborn back spasms in minutes, clearing asthma (no more inhalers), giving cancer patients with more energy, improving failing kidneys, improving dementia; I could go on. The list is long and you'll hear more stories throughout the pages of this book.

What motivated me to keep going is that I knew how much my own health problems affected my life and many people around me: my children, the rest of my family, my livelihood, my enjoyment of life. When a member of a family is ill, it's all about the illness rather than being a family. I was excited to watch people transform and enjoy their lives again, see families, couples, and children all thrive.

Spurred on by my initial successes, I continued to work with anyone who would let me for free to practice and learn. I developed new protocols to make up for any shortcomings of the material I learned previously and found they worked marvelously well. It seemed to make perfect sense as I imagine the cells with their structures, cell walls, nuclei, and organelles made up of the atoms and subatomic particles that are actually all just energy. They are brought around to full health by removing the energy of the cell that doesn't belong there, the part that is not in the energetic blueprint we are born with. In other words, the energy that causes the stress.

The true test of my ability to help people

Even though it seemed that many parts of my life had come together for me to be doing what I do now, I still felt unsure of this path. I am now what my former colleagues would poke fun at, how most of it was all in one's head, like the placebo effect. They snickered and laughed at "miracles" even if they didn't understand how those things came to pass. "It was just lucky!"

In the laboratory, if an experiment worked, it wasn't luck. If it didn't work, there was always a reason. This work is no different.

A scientist is something I felt safe being: experimenting then reporting results was straightforward and acceptable. It took a lot of courage for me to move out of that realm into one that doesn't have such clear physical explanations or boundaries. I knew that just like experiments in the laboratory, whatever affects someone's health/life/well being has good sound reasons for doing so.

As I was having these questions about my identity, I was given the biggest challenge anyone practicing a healing art could face. George, a family friend for 45 years, was in a coma after a bad traffic accident. His doctors said he would probably die shortly as his brain activity was low. I wanted to see if I could help George survive, but was terrified to try. It is one thing to ease pain, help someone sleep better, or even clear asthma from lungs, but to heal a brain crushed as extensively as his was is a frightening undertaking. I felt the weight of responsibility and it literally took my breath away.

On April 11th, I stood over George's bed in the ICU looking at the still, almost dead body of someone I've known since he was a child. It was surprising to see the face of someone I knew and didn't know. I grew calm and relaxed and felt a surge of resolve as I started working. I felt like I knew what to do before I knew what to do.

As I started to evaluate his condition, I saw he had the lowest life readings of anyone I had read to date, with a life force at 4%. His brain was massively damaged, he was hooked up to a variety of instruments with some of them ringing in alarm because his readings were so desperate.

I touched his hand briefly in order to connect to his energy field and to feel what was going on inside him. I began to adjust the energy fields around his brain by channeling "divine". Anyone can do this if they know what to feel for, a soft tickle on the skin, prickles in the palms, and an invisible resistance at the edges of the field. Certain types of energetic photographs and instrument readings confirm that what we feel is an accurate mapping of a persons energy field.

As I worked, the needles on the instruments around him began moving and the bells stopped ringing. I noted their readings and discovered later that the main dial was a critical indicator of brain damage, inter-cranial pressure. As I worked, the pressure reduced to one third its former value: I could see instrumental evidence of the adjustments I made on his energy field. Just like the inexorable pull of gravity, this invisible energy changed George's brain and the course of his life. I had no idea how I knew but I just knew that George was going to wake up.

I spent the next five days working on George from home, working for several hours. Things were going well for the first three days then all of a sudden, they started to get worse. I could tell that he grew weaker.

The cause soon became clear. The doctors had just told his parents to not expect him to wake up. There was no hope. When I had initially spoken to his dad, he was enthusiastic about my efforts. When the news came that his oldest son would die, he could no longer look upon George's face because of his deep pain. He separated himself from the hospital and visits.

His mother had the opposite reaction. She spent her days sitting by his bed, praying and being distraught that she was going to lose him. She blamed her husband that he no longer cared and arguments ensued in the days to come. As with other coma patients, George knew what was going on around him and decided that if the doctors said there was no hope, his dad no longer appeared, and his mother was sitting there distraught, then he better leave his broken body behind.
I didn't give up on him because I "knew" that he was going to be more than okay. I then checked him several times a day and boosted

his energy field back up so his body could heal. I could feel the changes happening within.

After this incident, it became very clear to me how important our words and actions towards others are to their wellbeing and health. Doctors need to be more cognizant of this. For no good reason, often a person slips away needlessly at someone's declaration of hopelessness.

I knew he would wake up on May 5th, our Greek Orthodox Easter, ironically the day of resurrection. Until then, I probed his condition every day and continued to correct his energy body.

On the sunny, warm morning of May 6th, the nurse came into the room to find George awake and alert. A few weeks later, he was home with his parents, having the best relationships he ever had with them, speaking coherently and getting better by the day.

I knew at once when this happened, that I was not only meant to continue this work and develop it further, but that I needed to teach it to others. After all, I am and have been for a very long time, a teacher at heart.

You can help yourself reach your highest potential.

I am not what one would call a miracle healer, a spiritual healer, or anything along those lines. I am more like an acupuncturist or masseuse. I don't wave a magic wand and poof, you get up and walk if you came to me lame. Instead, like the masseuse or acupuncturist, I help your body's energy field shift, sometimes rapidly or sometimes gradually, to allow your natural healing ability to proceed at an accelerated pace. I am not healing anything. Your body is doing that all on its own. I help you remove the internal conflict and stress.

Instead of all those "fluffy" titles, I prefer the term **scientific healer**. I possess no magical powers. In fact, you all come with the same equipment and can learn to do what I do.

We don't come with an instruction manual. I figured much of this out because I understand scientific principles, how energy fields work and how to change them. The principles are straightforward and in your scientific textbooks and research journals.

Much of what you learned of aging is a myth

It is clear from the hundreds of miracles that I've experienced on this life journey that our bodies were meant to regenerate in ways that we are only just beginning to understand. We've been told over and over again until everyone believes it is that aging is a downward spiral of desperation. That to stay alive you need to take a handful of medications every day or your heart will stop. We hear all the time that just because you are beyond a certain age you have to stop activities. Your career declines, you get weaker and frailer; that life belongs to the young.

This is a myth. If you manage stress by improving your energy and even fortitude, you will not age at the same rate.

You may or may not live longer but your quality of life will be beyond your wildest dreams. You never have to be ill again. You can go through your middle age and even old age without the typical cabinet full of medications for aches, pains, memory loss, tiredness, and lack of energy that is now considered the norm. You'll be able to do in your sixties and beyond what a strong healthy person in their twenties can do now.

All you need to do is learn how. Even though we are complex beings, this knowledge is straightforward and the exercises/practices fit into any busy schedule, aren't difficult to learn and consistently work no matter who you are.

Healing practice - Download the 15-minute healing audio and listen to it daily. http://scientifichealer.com/book-bonus/

Picture credit - Darren Hsu, 2013

2. How your energy changes with stress

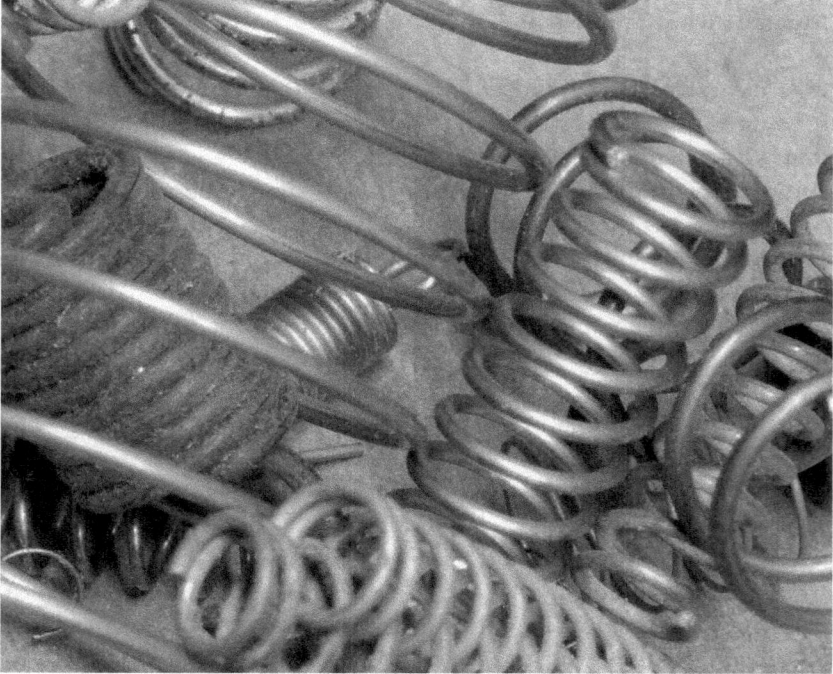

"Stress is the trash of modern life-we all generate it but if you don't
dispose of it properly, it will pile up and overtake your life."
Danzae Pace

As we've described in the introduction, all matter is energy, it has a measurable energy field, and the energy field of life reflects the perfect health blueprint plus the stresses added, whether mental, emotional or physical.

For the most part, medical schools have chosen to exclude the information in their curricula about our measurable energy fields as first discovered by Dr. Burr. As a result, most western trained medical doctors are ignorant of nearly 100 years of valuable data. Such information includes: our energy fields change long before illness or disease arrives, and that our fields interact with one another's.

An example of this might be when you are having an argument on the phone with someone, say, your parent. They are doing their usual thing with you, criticizing or disapproving the way you are handling something in your life. It makes you feel weak, lowers your energy.

Afterwards your mood is low, you can become angry or depressed and the outlook of your day just isn't the same anymore. You could be in France while your dad or mom is calling you from Indianapolis, Indiana. Your energy shifted by the exchanged words and feelings even though you were in totally different locations.

What if the words were praise, love, or an attaboy or attagirl for something you accomplished? Wouldn't you now be feeling elated, happy and grateful that you had such a supportive parent?

In each case, your energy was shifted even though you were in totally different locations. You are almost always interacting with your parent or child. You are part of them and they are part of you. Some people are estranged from their parents or children, but on some level you are aware of the other.

A way to shift your energy positively that you may have heard about is with laughter and comedy, as Norman Cousins did in his famous case. He published his book, Anatomy of an Illness, in 1979 to tell how he survived a potentially fatal illness through vitamins and laughter therapy. Praying for someone also shifts energy. Both therapies are under investigation by conventional hospitals and medical schools. The official stance as of now is that they do not help, although some hospitals have incorporated them into their healing programs. I also personally know several cancer survivors that they were helped by just such therapies. In any case, stress is reduced substantially, the strength of the body's field is improved and it promotes healing.

There are other means to raise your energy and reduce stress. If you listen to your favorite music, are you uplifted and feel happier?

What do you feel when walking in a beautiful location? How about after eating a healthy meal with your favorite people? Or when you've gotten a warm hug from a family member, a phone call from a friend you haven't seen in a while or a massage from a skilled masseur/ masseuse? It is clear that a two-way communication exists between your body and your spirit.

New studies show that putting your body in a stressful position, such as the fetal position, raises cortisol while standing tall and straight in an open position lowers cortisol. Amy Cuddy from Harvard University showed that just two minutes in an open stance such as straight with arms outstretched lowers cortisol by 20 % while it raises your testosterone by 20%. There are other indications of this two-way communication between body posture and your energy. Some counselors and psychologists found that a depressed patient gets better faster if you talk to him/her while walking. Motion makes you feel better. If you sit still too long, you will start to feel sluggish.

All of the positive actions raise your energy, make you feel better and keep you healthier. And there is so much more to it than that. This is exactly what I mean when I talk about working with people energetically to reduce their stress. Not only does shifting your energy fields directly help, but also the right words, actions, gestures, and interactions with others reduce stress, promote health, great relationships, and personal success.

The eight magical factors that keep you healthy

There are eight factors that keep you healthy. These factors have been identified over the last seventy years in medical research programs by such prestigious institutions as Yale, Harvard and Johns Hopkins. These programs sought out to discover what makes one person well and the other ill. What is it in their lives that kept them resilient and strong, healthy and living longer than average.

The most surprising of these results is that seven factors were more important than diet. Diet is important. However, you can still get ill even if you are eating a healthy diet, as I had.

These factors are explored throughout this book. Here I'll just describe them in brief.

These factors in order are
1. Relationships – loving and positive connection with others.
2. Healthy professional life – satisfying career that gives you pleasure and a feeling of self worth
3. Creative expression – an outlet that allows you to show your artistry in speech, writing, visually, audibly, motion, whether it's dance, singing, playing music, drawing, painting, sculpting, writing, poetry. Anything that lets you express you.
4. Spiritual connection – having a relationship with a higher power
5. Sexual connection – having a deep connection with another
6. Financial health – having a good relationship with money and having enough to sustain you and your family
7. Mentally healthy – brain and emotional health
8. Healthy body – eating right and staying fit

You will see in the following chapters that several of these factors need to be addressed to allow your body to heal. Others are things that you just need to do for yourself.

In my courses, I help you evaluate what I call an abundance wheel. This evaluation gives you a good idea what you can focus your time and energy into improving.

Now you'll see how you can interact with people even if they are not in the same location. Distance doesn't matter.

What is a quantum interaction?

People ask me all the time, how can we interact with one another if we are not even in the same room, building, city, state, or country as the other and we are not on the phone or connecting some other way electronically. There have been a number of interesting experiments lately related to quantum phenomena that show not only the possibility but the probability that all objects interact with all others.

First off, to make it clear, a quantum effect is a phenomenon that you only observe when you go down to atomic-sized dimensions. A few thousand molecules stuck together have very different bulk properties than something you can see with the naked eye in terms of size.

At atomic dimensions, you'll see things popping around with regards to their energy levels, you'll see that raising intensity doesn't do the same thing as changing the wavelength, and you'll see that electrons and neutrons have wavelengths and light can behave as particles. You'll also see that in order to understand fully how two particles interact, you need to account for them in all space, meaning even if they are infinitely far away from one another, they are still needing to be accounted for.

In the quantum world, scientists are discovering that even though several particles are not connected physically by any obvious means, perturbing one will also cause the others to move simultaneously. No obvious time delay occurs. It is as if they are all part of the same larger entity. This phenomenon has been called **quantum entanglement**.

For a scientist like myself that has studied these phenomena and solved the crazy looking and complex equations for a number of parameters, the term quantum healing sort of loosely describes exactly what is happening when one person affects the other's energy. I hear non-scientists use this term all the time often in the wrong context.

Really, it's our fields interacting with one another. The field around a heart can be felt up to at least 20 feet away. The fact that someone isn't in the same city or country doesn't seem to matter, there's something that seems to transcend distance, as if our fields can be extended via our connection to others.

Now that it is obvious you have a field, the idea that one person's energy field can affect another should not be so foreign to you. It is similar to when two magnets can interact. Every child knows this can happen if they have played with magnets.

But life is unlike inanimate objects. Your body has 9 trillion chemical reactions per day in each of its 38 trillion cells. You have miles of nerves and blood vessels, each transmitting either electrical impulses or matter through them. Your brain is sending trillions of signals running your entire being. Your heart is pumping continually with enough power to send your blood through your body rapidly and smoothly every minute of every day, and your muscles contract and relax all day long. All that activity creates several fields around your body. These fields interact with one another and with those of other people.

Unlike the interactions that I mentioned before, interacting fields transmit information even if you heard nothing verbal, tone or words, nor seen any facial cues/body language. For example, the field created by the heart is felt up to 20 feet away. You can enter into someone else's field, your mood could change and you don't even know why. You felt fine before you walked in. Look around, if this has happened, you may have noticed either a person that seems happy/content or sad/depressed. Do their emotions match up with what came over you?

I'm also sure you have experienced the invasion of your personal space when someone you don't know comes closer than about 3 feet to you. You automatically move away from that person if they do, even without being aware of it. It's as if there is an invisible sphere around you that needs to be clear in order for you to feel comfortable. When you are familiar and comfortable with that person, closer proximity becomes more comfortable. Unsurprisingly, the human field extends three feet from your body.

These fields are part of the fundamentals of energy medicine.

You already know a lot about energy medicine. Even medical insurance will pay for many modalities of it; these include massage, chiropractic, acupuncture, and psychology. In the personal development space, there is writing positive affirmations and making gratitude lists. Psychologists help people turn their thinking around, nutritionists help people eat better, and fitness coaches help people get moving. All of these also tame your stress, make you more resilient, improve your mental attitude and boost your energy.

These make up just a small part of energy medicine. There are structures and systems in the body that respond so well to positive energy that health can supplant illness, that happiness, energy, and joy can replace sadness and lethargy, rapidly and easily. You will learn about how to manage your energy here and just how powerful you all are.

I want you to entertain the notion that everything you read here is physically possible. In fact, not only is it possible, it happens every day whether you are aware of it or not.

3. Your energetic blue-print & the 7 stressors

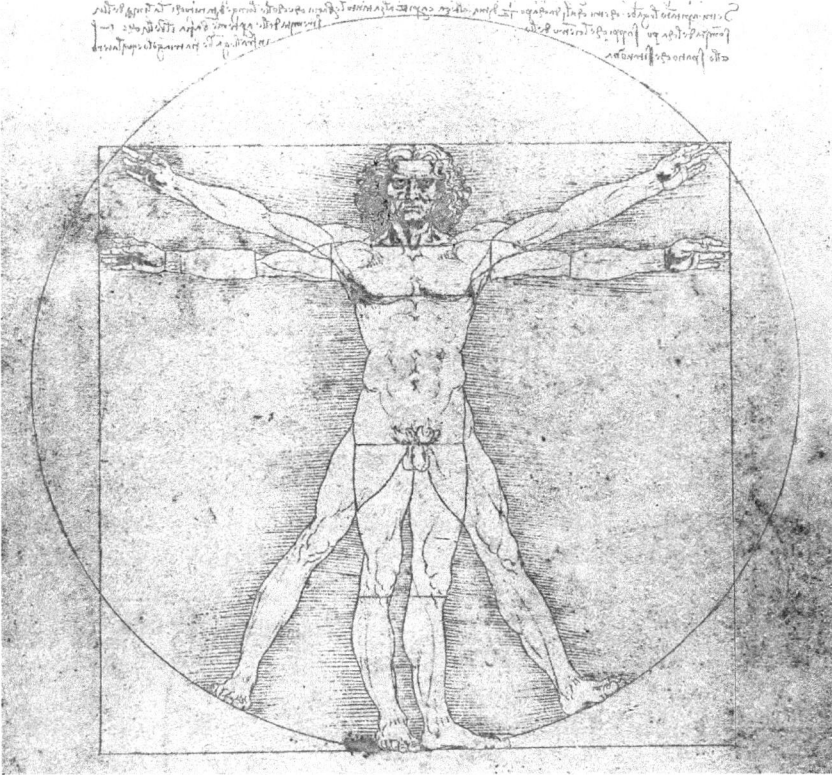

"Pressure and stress is the common cold of the psyche."
Andrew Denton

Traditional Western medicine practices seem to come down to "medicate or operate". You, the patient, are not to be trusted to help yourself so these more drastic and consequence-fraught choices are given you. Modern medical care, hospitalization and prescription medication is the third most common cause of death in the United States, following heart disease and cancer and the number one reason for filing bankruptcy and being destitute in "retirement". The best path is to not need medical care in the first place. I see that most people are simply unaware of what it takes to be healthy, even thinking that some of the modern so-called health foods are good for us.

Interestingly, if you once needed medication but have taken the necessary precautions to get healthier so you no longer need them, many Western medicine doctors are loath to take you off the prescription. In one such case, Bob, a relatively young man was on seven prescription medications. Even with good health insurance, this ran into the several hundred dollars a month cost not to mention the side effects that he was dealing with. Often, additional medication is prescribed to moderate the side effects caused by one of the original prescriptions.

Reducing stress and changing his body's energy a number of ways has weaned Bob off these medications with all his health parameters reading way better than average. He had to monitor his own blood pressure and blood sugar until they got so low that he had to reduce his medications. He also got off pain medication that he had been taking for decades for his back. The doctors didn't take him off the medications; he stopped taking them and went back to the doctor to see if he would prescribe them again. While this is not what is recommended you do, it is just an example of the typical behavior of Western trained doctors. There are wonderful doctors that will work with you: my strong recommendation is to find such doctor.

One further limitation of Western medicine is that it treats you for what is often the endpoint of a problem that began long before symptoms appeared. Without treating the root of the problem, the issue can develop into another physical ailment. For example, initial high cholesterol is an indication of inflammation; the liver sends out the cholesterol to protect you from this inflammation. Without treating the cause of the inflammation, a sustained high cholesterol level will usually lead to a statin prescription, which can translate into other problems, such as memory loss, muscular dysfunction, and diabetes.

The disappointing aspect of this "miracle medication" is that of the 100 million prescriptions of it in the USA, less than 1% of the people (under one million) derive benefit from it while 12% (12 million) are irreparably harmed, developing diabetes and muscle damage. This does not account for the people that feel just plain awful, lose their memory, and have no energy. Of the balance of these people, they are simply putting chemicals in their body that do nothing beneficial for them at great expense. Here the real heart of the issue is not addressed. As mentioned, the origin of the problem often begins with physical stress in the form of inflammation.

This fundamental concept of taking tests, dosing medicine or physical/talk therapy, and/or surgery is basically the toolbox MD's have been given to work from. Unfortunately, for many conditions, not only is it not enough, but people feel tired and listless and lose their brain vitality. Fortunately, there is help for everything and anything, as you will discover.

Next, I will show you the seven factors that affect our stress levels, then our existence, health, wellbeing, and happiness. You shall see that the origin of your illness or condition is not that simple. Instead, many more factors come into play than you would imagine and that conventional medicine only taps into a small portion of these issues.

You had an energetic blueprint long before you were born.

What many healers, both alternative and conventional medical practitioners, don't realize is that we all come with an energetic blueprint. I think this is one of the most important aspects of our existence. As you've discovered, this blueprint was first measured electrically by Dr. H.S. Burr in the 1930s and reported in several of his publications and books. He showed how the energetic blueprint starts at the fertilized egg stage and holds that information to adulthood. The size of the field is exactly the size of the adult and the alignment of the field on the fertilized egg exactly aligns with the spinal nerve and brain of the adult. This energetic blueprint also explains why our bodies maintain their integrity and don't grow off willy-nilly in all directions. This is true for all living things, both flora and fauna. One way to visualize the blueprint is by energetic photography (e.g., Kirlian photography).

This blueprint carries the information that you need to have perfect health. Dr. Burr showed the energetic body varies from the blueprint long before illness or dysfunction manifests itself. This means an energetic change takes place first, then the body later changes. It stands to reason that to remain healthy, realigning the energetic body to its perfect blueprint will circumvent illness and premature aging mainly because you are alleviating the internal conflict or stress on the body. Seven factors can create a deviation of your energy from your perfect blueprint, i.e., stress, leading your body to become ill and/or age prematurely.

The crux of the matter is that we are open systems, we take in food, air, water, information, and we expel them after we've got what we needed. We also interact with other people, and our environment, we have a family history, we have a tribal history, and we have a genetic line. And whether you believe this to be true or not, you have a past life that affects who you are now. It isn't absolutely necessary to believe whether you have a past life or not, only that this model works. It mitigates the problem if the energy of that influence is cleared and the stress dissipated.

In the Diamond Method protocol, part of the process of healing and rebuilding the body to a more youthful state is to activate the energetic blueprint and re-imprint it onto your physical body by releasing the causes of stress. This release removes the challenges on your body, which allows it to return to the parasympathetic or healing state.

The average experience is not an instantaneous healing, although tumors have disappeared overnight, but instead it sets a healing process in motion that continues for days, weeks and sometimes months to bring about a permanent healing. It takes consistency and a maintained effort, by both client and therapist/healer, once the stress release process takes place. To understand why a sustained effort is needed, imagine you decide to eat healthier so you manage that for one or two days, even a week, then go back to your old habits. You could not possibly expect a permanent and lasting change from two days or even a week of maintaining your healthier diet. The Diamond Method protocol is not magic: we all have access to the process, we are all capable of it. It's tangible, real, and easily sustainable. You already know many methods that will help your energetic body release stress and realign with your perfect blueprint. You'll discover many more in the pages of this book.

Here are the seven factors that affect your stress levels as you interact with yourself and your environment:

1. Your inheritance can affect you in surprising ways.

Your body is coded with three billion base pairs in your DNA, which is in every cell of your body. This includes a vast amount of information received from your parents. The way DNA carries information is coded using a brilliant three amino acid sequence along the DNA strands, meaning every cell has one billion words of coding in it.

DNA doesn't just carry information on eye color, hair color and even propensity for certain conditions. It will also carry inherited emotions, behaviors, body movements, likes and dislikes. It will carry tribal beliefs, family beliefs and even spiritual beliefs, all passed down from a parent or other relative. This is an emerging field of study called **epigenetics**. Only 5% of human DNA is involved in protein sequencing and synthesis, the rest is coded information that makes you you.

That these non-physical characteristics are inherited has been exemplified by a long-term study of identical twins that grew up separately, even without knowledge that the other existed. Their likes and dislikes were so similar, even down to liking to wear a lot of rings on their fingers, their favorite colors and foods. It baffled researchers that this happened; they eventually surmised that twins may have been connected in some way psychically. It may also be just coded into their DNA.

DNA ages as we grow older or abuse it. At the ends of the DNA strands are structures that have caught a lot of media attention lately: these are the telomeres. Telomeres start out early in life as long single stranded structures on each end of your double stranded DNA. They appear to protect the integrity of your DNA. The longer they are late in life, the more youthful your body. You can shorten the telomeres by abusing your body: drugs, smoking, alcohol, stress, lack of sleep, poor nutrition, poor hydration, no exercise. You can re-lengthen them to a certain extent by treating your body better, i.e., healthy food, no drugs, no smoking, no alcohol, exercise, rest, hydration, and practicing stress control.

There are two processes in the Diamond Method protocol that affect your DNA. First, these telomeres are re-lengthened so you become younger from the inside out. Second, the harmful epigenetic information that you have been encoded with is reprogrammed.

As an example of this, look at a family who has trouble with obesity. Is it eating and exercise habits? It can be but many times it is not. You'll see whole families still having trouble with staying lean. They all seem to look similar. We know that obesity is a health risk and it does not serve us well any more to be obese, where in prior times, the ability to hang onto extra weight was a good survival trait due to the feast and famine cycles before mankind began cultivating crops. So, here we sit with our awesome survival trait and it's harming us.

One part of Diamond Method protocol clears your DNA of these issues and gradually, the inherited issue dissipates from the body and the struggle to keep weight down is substantially eased. This is not to say that you can eat whatever you want and still be lean. This is a pipe dream. It does say that once you follow a prudent diet and exercise program, it will be effective rather than a struggle.

Karen is one such example. She said she wanted help with her type-2 diabetes and she wanted to be lean again. I worked with her for approximately two hours on three separate occasions reprogramming her body for leanness including removing her programming for obesity after menopause. Shortly afterwards, she spontaneously decided to go on a fitness regimen, changing her diet and exercise patterns. Nearly a year later, she is sporting a 40 lb lighter body and her type 2 diabetes is fully under control without medication.

Other issues that can be deprogrammed from your DNA include certain destructive behavior, ADHD, tendencies towards certain conditions or diseases such as Alzheimer's, arthritis, fibromyalgia, beliefs, etc.

Most of your DNA is a structural, biochemical marvel. It can carry millions if not billions pieces of information and usually the pieces not serving you any more only number in the hundreds.

2. Faulty self-beliefs shoot you in the foot

When you are born, you are not born with prejudices against yourself. You just exist, grow, and seek to survive. Babies are generally happy, smiling, and ready to take on the challenge of growing up.

It's the notions of the people in your life that you end up hearing, being told, and are taught that causes you to get in your own way. These notions could be prejudiced faulty notions that you see as your truth but aren't really factual. It's just your truth. Being open to possibilities beyond your own vision is the one of the most difficult things to overcome. Some of these limiting beliefs may be: that you're not deserving of more, that you're no good at relationships, that it's useless- nothing helps, that you aren't smart enough, good looking enough, lean enough, strong enough, or have enough courage to do what it takes to get past a certain point. Mostly this kind of self talk is based on what others have told you.

In the case of what others have told you, like a parent, a spouse, a sibling or a "trusted" friend, these messages can be more easily disconnected from our psyche because we've only incorporated them due to outside influences. This often requires the same kind of releasing of the negativity and stress that a relationship clearing entails. It also requires an emotional clearing, a simple releasing of the emotions that have lead us to accept those messages. One such message I heard as a child is that "You are so selfish, you'll never be happy when you grow up." It was sometimes a struggle to move past this message. These are things that a parent says in frustration or as an attempt to correct or modify your behavior, but are unaware of their lasting impact. While they might forget they said such a thing, you or your subconscious will remember it forever until you are able to work through it or release it.

Many coaches work through these barriers by not accepting what you say and pushing you to work through those limiting issues. The

Diamond Method protocol can assist in moving you past those barriers without all the talking and years of working through issues. The primary breakthrough occurs through identifying the concept or cause and releasing the energy or stress caused by it.

3. Your buried emotions

There are many ways in which you can come to storing emotions in your body. Many of the people I work with can recall incidents in their childhood that caused them to hang on to fear, anger, resentment, jealousy, anxiety, sadness, etc. A young child has difficulties processing their emotions during an early life incident and so the emotions get stored and locked into his/her body. Other people don't seem to remember any such incident. In such a case, I suspect they inherit the energy of that emotion, which gets locked up in the body, from one or both parents. You can imagine that anger resonates in a certain part of the body, say the liver. The liver of the fetus picks this anger up and the child holds onto it. Then you'll hear things like, "that child is just like his mother/father/uncle/aunt."

You have seen the manifestation of buried emotions: You know someone who seems to cry over the least little issue or someone who flies off the handle for no apparent reason. These are people that are carrying sadness or anger around who can be triggered by the least provocation. Anything that resembles the incident that caused the emotional pain in the first place, such as an unjust punishment, will incite the overreaction. Releasing these emotions is quick and easy without years of therapy or uncovering the reasons why they are trapped in us in the first place. These emotions can cause a lot of stress and even embarrassment and releasing them will be a big relief.

Here's where the issues can cross over from one of the seven areas of stress to another:
If you got angry with a parent a long time ago, it might color your relationships with that gender person the rest of your life. You can't enjoy people for who they really are; only what they represent to you. Releasing the anger from the body also shifts your perception of the gender in question.

4. Your relationship with yourself

When you are centered, you are being internally driven. This is what a psychologist or psychiatrist means when they tell you that you are centered. It actually refers to a physical phenomenon, where your energy field is aligned with your physical body. What does that mean, externally or internally driven, in practical terms? Here are some familiar examples: an externally driven life would be one in which you become a doctor or lawyer because you come from a family of doctors or lawyers and you are expected to follow the family business. Or it is to become a housewife with children because your parents said you'd never amount to anything and this was good for you. Their emotional reaction to you is projected into you and you internalize it. Until you realize this is their issue, not yours, you may be stuck with it.

An internally driven life leads to much less stress, more calmness, and a lot more happiness. You stop seeking approval from others for your behavior and need only look to see if you are satisfied with it. Your opinion will matter the most.

If you value yourself, you will also treat yourself better. You won't allow abuse of any kind, you will surround yourself with quality people that value you, you will feed yourself well with good foods, you won't seek out escapes such as addictions to substances or activities such as too much shopping, too much sex or substance abuse. Your life will be one of balance and feeling centered.

Breaking the energy stranglehold of external opinions and low self-esteem allows you to become more centered. Being centered leads to healthier relationships, healthier income, and healthier body. There are a number of exercises and protocols that address these issues specifically in the Diamond Method.

5. Your relationship with others

The quality of our lives depends on the quality of our relationships. We are social animals, we hang in packs, we interact within our pack or tribe, and our success depends on our success within the tribe. If we are good at enrolling people in our vision, we become successful business people, researchers, students, and have successful marriages.

Relationships that are plagued by stresses, anger, depression, illness, anxiety and phobias have a difficult time thriving. If these relationships are with people close to us such as our nuclear family members, it brings a lot of dysfunction into our other relationships. We can't fire our parents, siblings or other relatives. We can fire a spouse, but we should only do so after all other avenues of reconciliation have been exhausted. Why? Because your next spouse will be similar to the one you just fired until you figure out why you attracted someone like that and fell in love with him/her in the first place.

Many of you have gone into and out of a number of relationships if you have grown up in one of those dysfunctional environments. Each time you form or leave a relationship it leaves an energetic residue in your body, often referred to as relationship baggage. You have exchanged thoughts and emotions as well as physical touch with these people. An echo of their energy is in your body.

What do we do then? A Diamond Healing will clear out relationship baggage no matter what the source. The baggage can be from current relationships, former relationships and even people were abusive, strangers or not. If you have any emotion attached to that relationship, it can seem to have unfinished business. This can look like regret, anger, wishful thinking (wishing you didn't have to break up), anxiety or fear, or sadness. Anytime there is still an emotion attached to a past relationship, whether it is positive or negative, there's unfinished business and you are still in a relationship with that person. It means moving forward is more difficult if not impossible. The old ties hold you back.

Clearing the relationship consists of removing your energetic connection to those people and completing karmic contracts. It wipes the slate clean so to speak and allows both you and the other person to move on in a healthy manner.

Suzette had been angry over an old relationship for seven years. She was stuck. She was looking for a new relationship by going to online websites for singles but simply had trouble connecting. Her anger over the betrayal she felt with that old relationship just held her back. By releasing the stored up energy of that relationship in a four-step process that took approximately 15 minutes, she felt relief immediately, like a heavy weight had been lifted off her shoulders. Suzette hadn't realized that she never was out of that old relationship due to that lingering anger. She also didn't realize that because the anger she had stored in her body was apparent to others, it had affected her business adversely.

Once this energy and stress over her ex- was removed, her phone started ringing off the hook with new clients. Now she is busy with work and her fledgling business is thriving. While I have yet to hear of a new love in her life, Suzette was able to buy herself a new condo in exactly the location she desired. What clearing the old relationship did for Suzette was changing the focus on getting a new relationship to getting on with a satisfying and successful life. A new relationship will be arriving soon because nothing looks more attractive than a happy person.

As another example, I got divorced in 1994 and couldn't form a new healthy relationship because I was full of regret and sadness that this important relationship had ended. He was the father of my children and I admired and respected him although I knew that being with him was not healthy for me. When I finally did a clearing of his relationship and every other relationship I had, it became possible for me to again connect with someone on a very deep emotional level.

So even if it has been a long time between relationships, if there is an emotional connection of any kind to your former partner or family member, it will affect your future relationships, your health and your prosperity.

6. Your tribal beliefs

We were all born into a family first then a society. These groups carry their own belief systems, some good and some not so good for each individual. In general, we want to be accepted into our group. We feel ostracized and alone otherwise. This requires us to blend in. Even rebel groups have a belief system that can cause us to be excluded from it.

These belief systems give us a sense of belonging. Clubs are very popular: chess clubs, fitness clubs, stamp collecting clubs, rock hounding clubs, bicycle clubs, history clubs, etc. People love to get together when they have similar interests or political/religious beliefs. The amazing thing is that when one person is assertive at expressing his or her beliefs, others will join in even if they are not that adamant about it. They just go along to belong.

There are several of these tribal beliefs that don't serve us well. One such example was that women or other races are second-class citizens. It oppresses one group of people in favor of the other. This ends up creating conflict where none is necessary. Another such belief that I remember from school is that "girls can't do math," which excused every female child from even trying and the feeling that females were inadequate for many fundamental tasks. Other such beliefs are "boys don't cry", "you can't wear white shoes after labor day", "money is the root of all evil", "you have to work hard for your money", "the way to a man's heart is through his stomach", "Catholism (or whatever you are) is the one true religion", "You must be baptized or you are barred from Heaven", etc.

Each one of these is restrictive, disrespectful and/or demeaning. They lay down rules that are really unnecessary and in the long run hurt people and their relationships. A man that cries feels ashamed for having normal human emotions. A person who starts to get ahead starts sabotaging him or herself in order not to have too much "evil" money. Money isn't evil any more than a tree or water is evil. It's only energy and this is energy that could do a huge amount of good. The richest people typically establish foundations for helping the less fortunate. Don't you want to be one of those?

There are other group beliefs that also are harmful. They fall under the category of self-fulfilling. For example, it is said that the average life span of a human is approximately 80 years old now. People are gearing their lives towards that and set up their savings, their pensions, and their lifestyles to this goal. As the person's body ages, it will start to shut down as it approaches 80.

If a doctor gives you a prognosis that you will not live past 4, 6 or 8 weeks, generally the body will shut down and comply. If you make up your mind that you are a certain way or that a certain something will happen to you, it usually does. Our brains are fantastic computers and will set this in motion energetically and the physical will follow.

7. How your past lives can affect your future and beyond.

While many people will deny that we've lived before, there are many that accept this concept. It makes the most sense if you consider that our ultimate goal is to continue to learn and ascend along a path of higher consciousness or to a higher self.

Whether or not you subscribe to this concept, it is a model that serves to explain certain issues and helps solve problems that seem to have no root in the present life.
Remembering past lives is not generally useful as it distracts us from our tasks at hand. Besides, just like our memories in this lifetime, those will also fade over time. Our brains are generally not designed to remember and retain all incidents that happened to us because many of the events in our lives are simply not that important. It is the important memories that we retain consciously.

It is these important incidents that also may cause us to continue to run the programs forward into our future lives. For example, if you had a nomadic life in three or four of the past ten lives, you might feel the need to pull up roots often and move. This may harm your ability to form lasting and satisfying relationships.

Or if you had trouble with your lungs due to something like tuberculosis in a past life, you may have asthma in this life. The Diamond Method protocols can find and remove these influences systematically, allowing your body and spirit to be free of an influence that is actually harming you and bringing you poorer health, or keeping you away from a satisfying and lasting love connection or career.

Another serious influence from a past life that can occur is something like a time bomb. If you suffered a traumatic experience or a death at a certain age in a past life, when you become that age in this life, your health may crater for no apparent reason.

I've seen it occur a number of times and usually what happens is the spirit will slip out of the body and a similar incident will occur. If for example, someone died of a massive stroke at age 55 in a previous life, then in this life, at age 55, something happens that affects brain function and no one will be able to figure out the cause. Bringing them back into their body and removing the past life "time bombs" (and looking for others in several lifetimes) usually clears the problem. They may need further healing but it gets them out of danger of dying quickly.

One elderly person in perfect health went catatonic and was unrevivable. When I arrived on the scene, I saw his spirit was not centered in his physical body using the Diamond Healing protocols. I helped him re-center it and he revived a few minutes later. I found he had 4 time bombs in his past lives and removed them. A year later, no repeat incidents have occurred.

Nearly every current malady, whether it's spiritual, emotional, mental or physical could have a foundation in a past life. It is part of the process in clearing up the inner conflicts or stresses that cause a major dysfunction in your life, whether it's illness, career or relationships. More often than not, there is some indication of a former energetic influence that needs to be cleared before a healing can become permanent, which is the goal, of course, whatever the form.

There is one last influence that the scope of this book does not include, and that is that of outside spiritual influences. Western cultures do not embrace this idea although there is more airtime in shows about mediums, ghosts, and spirits from the "other side" than there has ever been. Many people view this as entertainment rather than reality, which had been my stance until relatively recently. These concepts can be left for future discussion for those that are interested in hearing the stories. I personally know three very talented mediums, two of which are seen on television. I'm sure the third will make her way there since she is an actress turned medium. One solves an FBI murder per week.

Spiritual outside energetic influence is of minor importance compared to the previous seven, especially considering how powerful we are as live beings. Recognizing that we command such power is the first step for manifesting what we desire in our lives.

In summary, your health at all levels is a manifestation of the seven energetic influences in your life. Some of these likely had nothing to do with your current life choices but were instead brought with you at birth. Your body will interpret these influences, if they operate contrary to your energetic blueprint, as stress: your adrenal glands will fire, sending you into the sympathetic or stress state. In this state, your body uses rather than replenishes your personal resources, tearing itself down little by little.

The Diamond Method protocols are designed to find these stressful influences and resolve them. As each stress or energetic pressure is released, a new balance is found until all the layers of stress are released. Each step brings you into the parasympathetic or healing state. While here, your body will replenish itself and heal, bringing you to your highest potential across all aspects of your life.

Homework: Today do something life affirming, whether it is taking a walk outside, writing down a list of things to be grateful for, writing down your assets (your personal attributes, something that you're happy you have), do some deep breathing or prepare yourself a nice healthy meal.

Reading: Dr. Candace Pert, The Molecules of Emotion. http://scientifichealer.com/molecules-emotion

4. Your energy body and how it knows the truth

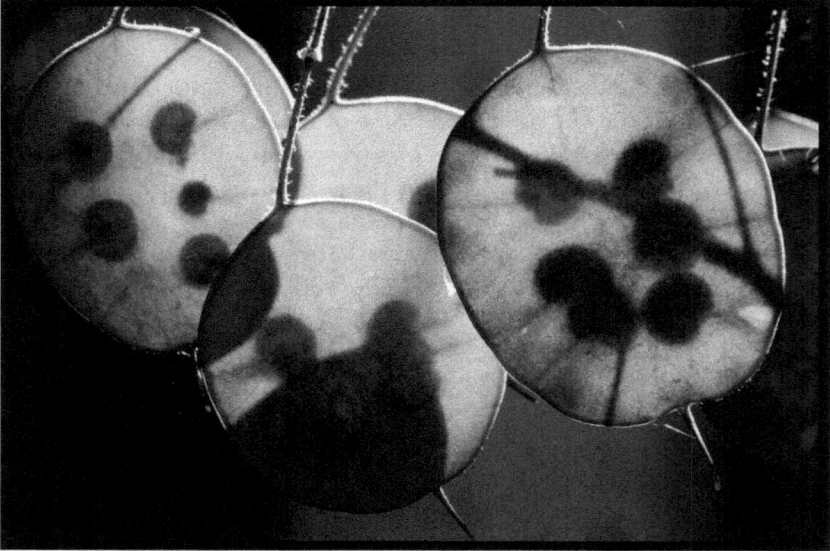

"Stress is an ignorant state.
It believes that everything is an emergency."
Natalie Goldberg

The energetics of agreement and disagreement

Imagine this: you just walked in the house and there's an argument going on and it has nothing to do with you. What is your reaction? Does your stomach churn or do you start to feel depleted and weak? You could have been having a good day and then you hear two people disagreeing and throwing a lot of negativity around. It immediately makes you tired and drained. This is a natural reaction.

On the other hand, if you walk into your home and someone has surprised you by having a meal prepared or cleaning up your house, your energy goes way up and you feel lighter than air for quite some time. Your strength goes up.

Telling someone you love them makes them feel stronger and

increases their energy. Being angry with someone depletes their energy and even their strength. This is no accident. The energy field in your body responds to your psyche. When you feel supported, cared for, loved, heard, accepted, or even agreed with, your strength increases: yes, your physical strength. And the opposite occurs when you feel disapproved of, yelled at, hated, ridiculed, cursed at, ignored, or even disagreed with. This is one of the reasons the quality of your relationships and your language with yourself and other people are so important.

The energetics of agreement and disagreement are even more profound. Our body field reads the fields of everything around it, including interacting with the fields of those people around us. If you are not schooled in how to dissipate the negative energy, you will absorb and keep it. Yes, we all have this ability, we are all built with the same equipment and our bodies work as receptors of a sort, much like your eyes see and your ears hear.

Your body senses the energies around it. You were meant to do that. Even if you don't have one iota of "psychic ability", you can determine things that are true or not true by practice. The first thing you need to discover is how are you going to ask your body whether something is a "yes" or a "no." You have a very powerful lie detector built into your nervous system: some people refer to it as a b.s. meter. Your body works much like a computer, with 1's and 0's, with "1" being yes and "0" being no. Your body regulates all the systems in the body in this manner.

A "yes" makes you stronger. If you are in sports, you know that positive self-talk and positive encouragement from a coach can vastly improve your performance. Either you or someone else believing you can achieve something can help you realize that achievement.

A "no" weakens you. If you hear "no" all the time, you may end up depressed, tired, having no energy. You won't be able to kick yourself into overdrive to do something spectacular.

This is the premise of discovering your "yes" and "no". All questions need to be phrased so the knowledge you seek can be discovered using this simple test.

Behavioral kinesiology: your body doesn't lie

This phenomenon is well known amongst alternative health care workers and is used to test all sorts of issues. It was first brought to attention through the work of Dr. John Diamond in his book "Behavioral Kinesiology". He found through experiments that we humans test strong and weak with several universal symbols. The testing muscle is usually the deltoid (shoulder muscle) and the tester will request you to hold your arm out from your body and test whether looking at something, touching something (to test for food and environmental allergies), or reacting to a situation makes that muscle go weak or strong. The stronger you test, the more that question, symbol, or food, etc., agrees with you. An example might be, while holding some peanuts at your waist level (more about that in a minute), "Is this food at least 70% good for me?" If you test weak, you should avoid peanuts on that day.

Dr. David Hawkins has reported in his books how he spent years doing muscle tests on thousands of people showing the reliability and consistency of muscle tests. The basic difficulty is separating the emotional attachment from the result, as you'll see shortly.

This yes-no response is one that will allow you to discover things about yourself (or others) without being in the least bit "intuitive" or "psychic".

Using your arm's deltoid muscle by yourself isn't always practical. When I first started using this technique 20 years ago, I would use a big bottle of water and lift it to my side (easy to lift is "yes" and hard to lift or even no lifting "no"). I would do this in the grocery store and other places to test whether I was allergic to something. I developed a more convenient test later: you'll see that in the next section.

Later, I put various foods in packets so I couldn't tell what they were, numbered them, and picked them up without looking to see if I was influencing the results. After all, there are certain things that you think you "love" and don't want to give up because your body says "no". Being prejudiced for it and happy to look at it because to you it's yummy, such as dark chocolate, CAN influence the results (you chocolate lovers know who you are). I systematically tested every few days to see if the results changed during the natural monthly cycles. They did. (This result corresponds with the observation that the immune system subsides during ovulation so the body doesn't kill any potential babies before they can be formed.)

Your simple yes/no test, your path to discovery

Lifting a big bottle or having someone push on your arm isn't always practical. You need something fast and easy because in working with energy, you will be asking a lot of questions of yourself. This is going to be your primary access to discovery if you are not a "psychic" or intuitive type. It takes practice and patience to develop this. It is a process that you should use every day, even if it is only to ask your name: "Is my name _____?" You could also ask silly questions as one of my medium friends does, "Am I wearing a pink tutu?" If your energy is blocked in some way or you are not all the way back into your body, your own name will produce a "no" result and a "yes" answer to an absurd question. Just using your hands in some way is ideal.

You <u>can</u> prejudice the results based on your personal preference. This is why practice is needed, so you can learn to detach from the result. Adopt Einstein's philosophy. After being asked how he felt about so many people trying to prove him wrong, he responded that he had no interest in being right, he just wanted to know whether or not he was.

Knowing the correct answer, the unprejudiced one, will give you a starting point for healing, stress relief, correction, and improvement. If you don't allow the correct answer to come because you won't like it if the answer is "no," then you can go on for a long time with a dire situation making your (or someone else's) condition worse. You don't want to be eating foods you are allergic to because damage continues to occur, shortening your life unnecessarily. Many allergies CAN be corrected, so knowing IS important.

The yes/no test needs to be fast, convenient and doable even in tight spaces. To this end, a finger-based test is ideal. Anyway you can imagine to test a muscle as strong or weak and it works consistently for you is the right one. There is no right way or wrong way, only the way that works for you.

Here are a few of the finger based tests taught by various practitioners:

Intertwined fingers: make loops with you index finger and thumb on both hands. Intertwine the loops and try to pull apart. If you have resistance and it stays together, it's a yes; if it slips apart, it's a no.

Left index finger pressing on right ring finger: it accesses the triple warmer meridian that ends at the end of the ring finger. This is a preferred method by some healers. The right ring finger will flop or go loose on no.

Pressing the fingers of your opposite hand together, i.e., form a spider on a mirror (you get the idea) and press. If the fingers give way, it's a no. I have gotten so used to the response for yes and no, it only takes a millisecond to determine the result.

In any of these tests, you don't need to press so hard that after a few tests you experience muscle fatigue and can't test any more. You just have to determine if there's resistance or not. A light touch will do.

A pendulum also works. Ailene, one of my students, calls her pendulum her business partner. She told me during one of my course sessions that the way to do this is to stand and let the pendulum drop in front of your body. Ask the pendulum to show you a neutral. This is usually still. Then ask for a yes and watch what it does. It might be a clockwise circle or a wagging back and forth towards and away from your body. Then ask for another neutral. Do the same for determining the no. Some of you may find this an easier method but after asking hundreds of questions in a day because sometimes I'm on the phone several hours a day working with clients, I would take five times longer to discover how well the various parts of the energy (and physical) body are functioning. Just one reading of basic 19 parameters can includes hundreds of yes-no tests. There may be a way to shortcut this using a pendulum, but finger tests are great for speed.

Now that you have this seemingly magical way of discovering the truth about something, you need to practice and practice a lot.

What should you practice on?

When you wake up in the morning, ask yourself, "am I [your name]?" Put your own name in the blank. Why would this not always be a yes, you are probably wondering? This is indicative of a number of things. One, you may not be entirely back down into your body. Remember, you are not your body. You are your energetic essence, your spirit, your soul. Your body is just a physical manifestation of that. It's the computer; you are the operator. This would tell you your first thing to do in the morning. Two, your channels may be blocked, that means you need to clear them before you can even get a yes for your name; you'll learn about these channels shortly. Or three, you may be dealing with spiritual parasites that need clearing. You can determine which of these are causing your "no" response through a series of steps that I'll talk about in the next chapter, but you now get the idea that this is powerful.

The next thing you can practice is asking the obvious questions and seeing how your body responds to them. Keep testing until you feel those answers are consistent. It can be anything that has an obvious yes/no component.

Then you can move on to the less obvious questions. If you know someone well, you can connect with his/her energy (just think of them) and ask questions about them. Warning, don't tell them any answers without their requesting it. It is an invasion of privacy. I would stick to the obvious kinds of things such as height, hair color, age and so forth and don't pry.

This is such a powerful tool in your hands: use it only for the good of yourself and others, not for "power". I've not seen lottery numbers ever reveal themselves ahead of time amongst any of us that do this kind of querying, in case you were wondering. The karma you take on in either invasion of privacy or gambling may make your life extremely difficult.

Authenticity and Integrity

If you now realize that truth strengthens your body, you will also realize that anything that is out of integrity with yourself will weaken you. This includes the little lies we tell ourselves and sweep under the carpet so we don't have to face them head on.

Little things might be something like looking at yourself from the neck up so you don't have to face that you've gained weight. Another might be a lie of omission for something that needs to be told. That is not something that would hurt the other person, just a missing fact such as not telling someone you've been married before when you're about to get married. It could be misrepresenting your age on a dating website or taking your picture from the waist up although you have big hips.

There are a number of people that stretch the truth, not realizing that this is out of integrity and weakens them. Each time you tell the truth, you gain strength. It might even be that you say you're going to be somewhere at a certain time, such as a doctors appointment. Doesn't it upset you that the doctor keeps you waiting? Their office is out of integrity. I get up and leave if I have to wait longer than 15 minutes or look for appointment times with the least amount of lag time.

Have you ever been to conferences and events where the schedule was so loosely held that everyone in the room grows irritated? That's because the organizers are out of integrity and not respecting the time of the participants. It is common that you will return from such a meeting totally exhausted because you are holding their space for them while they are not holding their part of the bargain.

In any relationship, openness and truth strengthens the relationship while being secretive weakens it. It is a good habit to get into to speak the truth. You'll see that one of the major energy channels will clog up if you habitually stretch the truth no matter what the situation.

In the next section, you'll learn about the spiritual body and what to test on yourself. It will also explain what to do if the answers are less than ideal.

Reading: Dr. John Diamond, "Behavioral Kinesiology"   http://scientifichealer.com/body-doesnt-lie

Photo: the honesty plant

5. How your spirit fuels your body for great health

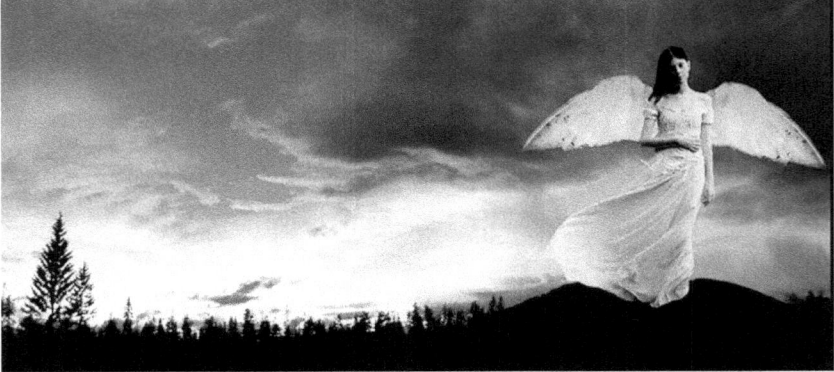

"Worry is worthless. It can't change the past or control the future. It only spoils the moment."
Darrin Patrick

You may have heard this before, that we are spiritual beings on a physical journey and not a physical being with a spiritual component. The spirit is you, your essence, your intelligence that is not in your brain, what you came into life with, what fuels your physical body and what you leave with once your physical body is spent. It is the part of you that survives past the physical realm. Nearly every world religion has similar stories and concepts.

Once the spirit inhabits a body, there are several energy structures that appear and only exist while the body is alive. Once a person dies and the spirit leaves the physical body, these structures dissolve. These include energy channels and openings as well as the fields surrounding the body/spirit combination.

Why hasn't modern medicine embraced these ideas, which have been around for millennia? Instrumental evidence has been around for a century. It doesn't make sense since there has been so much evidence for working with fields/channels, such as in acupuncture or homeopathy, and they're as effective or more than medication or surgery. Even on such sites as Wikipedia, you'll read that many "alternative" health practices are "quackery". I have often asked myself why this is labeled quackery while standard medicine such as statins for lowering cholesterol is not, given that they only marginally improve the longevity for 1% of those taking it while it harms 12%.

Let's say, for the moment, that our spirit, that energy that is us, does occupy our physical body. This concept could explain the many issues not curable by conventional medicine. Take, for example, the term "being centered." When you are centered, you are being internally driven; this is what a psychologist or psychiatrist means. In our model, it also refers to a physical phenomenon. The spirit is anchored to us physically through the pancreas, which symbolizes the sweetness of life energetically.

When you are not centered physically, your spirit is out of alignment with your body. The body is like a computer. A computer can't run properly unless there's an operator or programmer. It's just a machine and we become an animal without our spirit. The spirit needs to be attached physically in the body to animate us.

When the spirit is not centered, and it usually is not, a whole host of things can happen. We as a society in this day and age tend to pull our spirits up towards our heads. We are very cerebral. When that happens, there is too much thinking and not enough acting. People that are thinkers do a lot of sorting. They sort the information, their behavior, the behavior of others, their interactions, their desires, etc. It slows their reactions and they become fearful of decisions instead of acting and moving with confidence.

The further up the spirit is pulled, the further off center we become. It also affects our physical body. In most people, it stops at the hip. These people tend to develop lower back problems and knee problems simply because that part of the body isn't being fed properly on an energetic level. Some spirits will be pulled up to the waist, where lower digestive issues tend to arise. Others will have it at the shoulders where heart/lung issues tend to be a problem.

Pulling the spirit back down into the body can wake someone up that's groggy or sleepy. At a meeting recently, Alison told me that she was afraid of her long drive home due to grogginess. One wave of the hand brought her back to full alertness and she was able to get home safely. Alison later told me that her long drive home went without incident. Brenda mentioned that right after I pulled her spirit into balance, her brain fog vanished. One of my students, Karen, mentions that the simple act of pulling herself down into her feet every morning cleared the leg pain she's experienced for several years.

A measure of how well the body and spirit are integrated is the life force reading. The lower the life force, the more ready that person is to leave for good (in other words, die). Remember, George, my comatose family friend? His reading was 4%: the doctors gave him no chance of surviving because he had no obvious brain activity. By raising his life force reading, sometimes several times a day, he was able to survive because it allowed his body to heal. As a note, his life force dropped precipitously when his mother sat at his bedside and cried all day she projecting what the doctors had told her. He gave up even while he was in a coma. As a healer, I had assured him that he would recover completely and be able to overcome his old challenges. And it has been so.

If the spirit is somewhere above the neck and only occupying part of the head, you will find people somewhere on the spectrum of autism or ADHD. These people tend to exhibit a disconnect between the body, the emotions, and the mental body (thinking, brain). Any part of the body can be excluded, whether it's the eyes (and these people seem to not see things as others do), the mouth (inappropriate language will shoot out of the mouth), or a single limb. When you engage any of these people in conversation and you talk about body awareness, you'll find that they've disassociated parts of their physical self from who they are. Nowhere does any sort of conventional medicine or even most alternative treatments handle this sort of disconnect. Conventional training takes years and is emotionally/financially taxing on the family.

You'll often meet people extremely off center where they are not able to visually see what you are seeing and they will look at something and not be able to react emotionally to it the same way you would. For example, an autistic child will not be able to process a smiling face or outstretched hand as a friendly gesture. Or if they do, they often don't react to it physically by returning a smile or commenting in a friendly way.

A healthy human existence requires the spirit to be centered in the body, the same thing a psychiatrist would say about a healthy psyche. One of the first procedures completed during the Diamond Method protocol is getting you centered. Most people report a feeling of lightness or rightness when this happens. They relax, move out of stress, and move into ease or into the parasympathetic system. I've seen autistic children and adults become more fluid in their speech and see emotions play across their face inside of a half an hour. Their bodies seem to work better, less cramped with more fluid movement. This in itself is a miracle; every baby should be pulled into their body as they are born, which can be done by touch, massage, being held and bathed as well as energetically. I have done this and watched these children grow and develop at an incredible pace into healthy young children. This in itself is very exciting.

Paul, a 14-year-old high functioning autistic child was brought to me by his mother. He suffered from digestive problems, his hips did not engage when he walked, giving him a stiff and halting gait. His face remained passive and emotionless while in conversation and he answered most questions with single word answers. His interests varied little, he only watched the history channel and spent most of his free time building one type of model ship. He was able to attend conventional schooling as his intelligence was well above average. He even sought to do activities with other children his own age.

After a half an hour work with him, while engaging him in conversation about his likes and dislikes, I helped center his spirit in his body and reactivated his energy channels (which are mentioned in the next sections of this chapter), his face started to show his underlying emotions. He walked more smoothly and he started speaking in sentences. After 4 sessions, he went back to the doctor who referred Paul to me and it was discovered that his digestive health had improved dramatically and the number of supplements and medications necessary for good health could be substantially reduced. He now was much more verbal and articulate, speaking in paragraphs instead of single words, while showing more emotion on his face.   He expressed his likes and dislikes with much more emotion in his voice.

Children under the age of 20 are relatively easy to work with as they have spent a lot less time in inner conflict.   They seem to take to being centered and balanced much more easily.   However, the centering and awakening can happen at any age.   Clive, a 27-year-old man, had suffered rejection and difficulties in school his entire life.   He too has a form of autism known as Asperger's syndrome. He had emotions that he showed regularly, often represented by bursts of anger, causing people around him to shy away or shun him. Down deep, Clive was a sweet man and wanted to make his own way in life and stop being dependent on his parents.

After three fifteen-minute sessions of centering, opening and realigning the energy systems in his body, he startled everyone around him by being cheerful, helpful and kind to those around him. He was able to find and retain employment.   His own parents didn't recognize him.

Many high functioning people with Asperger's or autism are actually able to stay in jobs, many of which don't require them to interact with others much. This might include researchers or lab workers. Social interactions are often difficult for them.   Improved social interactions would increase their chances of success as it did for Clive.

Now that we've seen how the spiritual body needs to be centered in the body, there are several energetic structures that form in the body when we are born.   These energetic structures correspond to physical structures in the body, including nerve endings, polypeptide and endorphin receptors.

Your energy channels feed specific areas of the body.

There are a huge number of channels, some say thousands, but there are 72 major openings that bring energy in from the outside to feed our physical body.   The channels absorb energies from our environment, from other people, and other life forms.   The locations correspond to major nerve nexi from the spinal cord and major receptors. These major receptors, including endorphin, polypeptide, and other hormonal receptors, align along the meridians of the body as mapped out for acupuncture.

There are seven main channels along the medial line of the body, down the center of the head and torso, front and back. In the eastern culture, these are known as chakras. There are also minor openings on the joints, like elbows, knees, wrists, ankles, and hips. We also have minor openings at the eyes, ears, breasts, feet and hands. The channels need to be open and collecting energy in order for our bodies to be healthy. They can shut down when they are overwhelmed with a stream of negativity, such as deceit, anger, jealousy, or evil. It works much like the iris of the eye closes when the light that strikes the eye becomes too bright and too much for the sensitive eye receptors. A sustained stream of negativity will close down the openings chronically, causing certain areas of the body to be starved of energy.

You close down your energetic channel to stop the negative influence from entering your body and wreaking havoc on your insides. If you are in a constant state of bombardment, say in a dysfunctional job, family or situation, the blockages can become more or less permanent fixtures in our energetic bodies. Sometimes you are even born with a blockage because your family of origin had it in abundance.

Using the Diamond Method protocol, the blockages can be quickly opened allowing the flow of energy again. With each clearing, I get remarks from clients that they've not felt that energetic or that good in years; that they want to do things again.

You were probably never taught how to clear the blocked channel directly. In fact, most people aren't even aware that they have these blockages and have no idea how much better they can feel and function, never mind how much healthier they can be.

We are all aware of actions we take that do make us feel better.

Some of these actions might be listening to music, doing something creative, exercising, getting plenty of rest, eating healthy food, being around nurturing people, working through an issue via talk therapy, or even cleaning your house. Do these sound familiar? They should, they are some of the eight drivers for good health as discovered over decades of research from top medical schools in the country as mentioned in the last chapter.

Clearing a blocked channel is a simple procedure that anyone can learn. One method is to listen to a relaxing meditation that helps guide your body to keep your channels open. Go to http:// diamondhealingmethod.com to get yours.

I've watched swollen and inflamed joints calm and shrink in a matter of fifteen minutes by opening up the channels in the joints and apply healing energy to them. Pain relief from arthritis, back pain or fibromyalgia is usually achieved. Bob from an earlier chapter suffered for over 40 years with back pain. Realignment of the spirit, opening the main energy channels and the channels along the back stopped the pain dead in its tracks. The following day, I ran an allergy assessment and found that gluten was a problem. Not only is this client pain free and off a forty year long series of pain killers, but the excess belly fat dropped off at a breakneck pace. Bob is over 50 lbs lighter in six months time and his other middle age symptoms have also dropped away as the body is now being fed energetically. This alone saves him over $900 per month in medications.

Acupuncture, chiropractic and massage are common alternative medicine practices that help open up the energy channels. The Diamond Method uses a slightly different but equally effective method that you can apply to yourself, which you will discover later in this chapter.

The role of the 7 major energy portals in our human survival:

Our major energy portals are aligned along the medial line of the body front and back, top and bottom. There are seven of them and correspond physically to a set of nerve nexi and major body receptors, including endorphin and polypeptide receptors, discovered by recent biological researchers such as Dr. Candace Pert. Dr. Pert discovered that these receptors aligned along the meridians and medial line of the body as part of her thesis (supervised by Dr. Solomon Snyder).

Nerve networks from the spine ended in these major medial portals, showing that these areas are physical receptors. Energetically, they are receptive areas that fuel various parts of the body. These are outlined below. There are also ideal colors that these portals seem to carry but these colors are not unique. They are normally depicted as a rainbow, moving from lowest energy colors to highest energy colors as seen in the image below. They can be a range of colors. Depending on which gender you are, some will serve you better than others.

These rainbow colors are not necessarily the healthy ones that a clairvoyant might see. It is said that each of our energy bodies, that is, the spiritual, emotional, mental and physical bodies each have their own system of energy channels or chakras to feed those areas. There are layered above the physical body and may have admixtures of the various layers showing up. In the following sections, these colors are mentioned.

The seven major channels/chakras, and some minor ones including those in joints and hands and feet, are described in the following: with their function, location, and ideal colors. Except for the one on the crown, all portals appear conical, with the narrow part of the cone closest to the body and expanding outward away from the body. On the crown, it appears more cylindrical rather than conical. For the chakras/portals on the front of the body (2 through 6), there is a matching one in the back.

These portals need to be open, spinning and active for you to enjoy perfect health. The spinning can be imagined much as the flow of current in one direction along an electrical wire produces a field that rotates about it. If you were to place the thumb of your right hand along the direction of current flow in a wire, your fingers would indicate the direction of the field, which is known as the right hand rule in physics. Put your right thumb towards your body, your right fingers point the way to the direction of spin of your energy portal.

These portals feed the various glands, organs and systems in the body in their proximity, which is listed below. As mentioned in the last section, there are a variety of reasons why they might not be on and functioning properly, from emotional reasons to disease, injury and past life issues. A Scientific Healer can help open them back up and get them moving again and so can you. During any healing session, it is usually the first thing that is checked and made active again.

Some healers suggest you close your chakras down when you are in a situation with someone or something that is an energetic threat and could deplete you, as mentioned in the last section. However, that doesn't need to happen if you learn how to protect your field edges with an energetic barrier that blocks low energy thoughts, emotions, and intent. You will read more of that at the end of the chapter.

What is the importance of colors of the portals? While for the most part, once your energy ports are opened to allow healing energy to enter the body and energize it in the various locations, the color that's established is healthy for your needs. It might not always be the same each time. In most diagrams, you'll see them established as increasing in frequency from the base of our spine up to the crown of our heads. There are also, according to many schools on the spiritual body, many layers to your field or aura as well as many layers to the portals or channels. The different layers can be different colors depending on the spiritual connection.

As we change and grow and move through our life, our main energy portals will appear as different colors, become damaged, and even be closed off entirely. The connections need to be reestablished and reenergized to enable great health and a feeling of wellbeing.

To open and energize any portal, intend for it to be open while you are moving your hand as if you are clearing out anything in the way: a scooping motion in the direction of the spin (usually counter clockwise). Extend your fingers and move your hand around at the wrist. First clear the front then move to the back.

If just your intent is not clear enough for you to focus on, you can imagine your energy body in front of you as if a mini version of your body is before you. It is an energetic representation of you. This works well because your subconscious works very symbolically. You apply the rotating scooping motions to the energy body you imagine in front of you. You keep going until you muscle test 100% open for each portal or chakra.

Your root portal fuels survival.

The root portal (first chakra) supports our survival, such as eating, breathing and supporting ourselves financially. It connects us to our tribe or family, and is the foundation of our emotional and mental center. Organs associated with the root include muscles, bones, hip joints, spine, blood, and immune system.

Spiritual and emotional issues that can block energy into your root include knowing when to feel safe and secure in the world, knowing when to trust or mistrust, knowing when to feel fear, and finding a balance between independence and dependence. Physical dysfunctions that can occur as a result of a closed down root portal are: back pain, scoliosis, rectal cancer, fibromyalgia, arthritis, and skin problems. These problems also appear when the spirit is not fully engaged in the body.

The root chakra is pointed down from the base of our spine and provides the energy of birth and death and energy to the legs allowing us to be able to move.

In practice, I see low energies on root chakras when someone is not sure whether to stay or leave life. Sometimes, the ability to support oneself financially is compromised. If it is off, completely closed down, it is usually at the beginning of the end.

Good colors that support your survival at this portal are:

Red: In this chakra, red provides capacity to be and to exist. Red in the root or base chakra provides energy and action.

Green: Green provides a driving force for wealth and can also promote happiness. Green is less balanced than red because the focus is primarily on wealth rather than survival.

Pink: Pink in the root chakra energizes the capacity for love. This color works better on average for women than men, especially since this chakra is "male" in nature.

As you can see, red, the color normally depicted for this portal, IS a good color for it to be. Green and pink are also healthy colors although less so. This is not the case for many of the other major portals.

The Sacral Portal supports creativity in the arts as well as reproduction.

The sacral portal supports your creativity in the arts and sensuality/sexuality for women, finances, personal power, relationships and pleasure. This portal is feminine and receptive. Organs associated with this second portal include uterus, ovaries, vagina, cervix, large intestine, lower vertebrae, pelvis, appendix, and bladder.

Spiritual and emotional issues that can block energy in the sacral portal are balancing your drives toward sex, money, and relationships; co-creating with others; defining boundaries; and struggling with when to give and take and when to be assertive and passive.

Physical dysfunctions that can occur are: lower back pain, sexual impotency, urinary problems, and appendicitis.

Fine artists and dancers are fueled by this energy source: the manifestation of this type energy is seen in the creativity of painters, sculptors, jewelers, dancers, musicians, and lovers.

In practice, low energy in the sacral area shows up with people that are in the midst of relationship stress such as divorce. I had tried to pull the spirit back down into Judy when she said she was feeling off the ground and off center. I immediately hit a block at the second chakra. When I asked if she had relationship issues, she mentioned that she was in an ugly divorce. The energy of that relationship needed to be removed before her energy (and her spirit) could flow past it. After removing that emotional hindrance, Judy said she felt more at peace and felt centered again.

Often clearing out your old relationship issues will improve your financial situation. Louise reported a 30% increase in income from clearing out anger towards her father. She did not change any other behavior, such as advertising or marketing. People just perceived her differently, felt the energetic shift and were more attracted to her.

As you can see, both love and money are related to your sacral chakra.

Other maladies that appear due to low sacral chakra activity are endometriosis, fibroids, infertility, dysmenorrhea, PMS, incontinence, and UTI.

Good colors for this portal that support physical creativity are:

-**Pink,** the color of divine female love and is better for women at this portal.

-**Green**, the color of divine male love but is also good for women here. Green provides fuel for a healthy, creative life as well as health and vitality.

-**Red,** the color of passion, intention, enthusiasm and drive.

Orange is the color normally depicted on figures and in books as healthy for this energy portal but orange is less desirable than the three colors above.

Solar Plexus Portal supports your will

This portal provides energy for your personal will and for the development of your personality, self-esteem, and ego. It is located right above your belly button front and back. When you have a fully healthy will, accomplishment and fulfillment are very much supported. It propels visionaries to heights most people find unattainable. Once your solar plexus is feeding you well, you'll find you're able to manifest more for yourself.

Since your root provides for sexuality for men and your solar plexus provides compassion and power, a combination of the two drives male sexuality. For both genders, the solar plexus feeds the small intestines, liver, gall bladder, stomach, kidney, pancreas, spleen, adrenal system, middle spine and 80% of the cellular body. What that means is that your solar plexus is providing energy to a majority of your cells and provides you with a strong life force.

Spiritual and emotional issues that can block energy in the solar plexus are challenges with self-confidence, self-respect, competence and skills in the outer world, substance abuse, aggression, defensiveness, making decisions, and competitiveness. Physical dysfunctions that can occur are: ulcers, irritable bowel syndrome, heartburn, diabetes, diarrhea, indigestion, anorexia, bulimia, and hepatitis.

The solar plexus plays a large role in outer world accomplishment and wealth building.

Good colors for this energy portal: For both genders, **green** provides strength, health, and wealth while **red** provides force and vitality.

In some portal layers, yellow is *not* as good of a color as this is often associated with mental energy and our will is best served with the primary colors of green and red for reactivity, energy, and vitality rather than mental energy.

Your solar plexus portal spins in front counter-clockwise and in back clockwise.

In my healing practice, I see a lot of adrenal fatigue and low liver function. As mentioned earlier, up to 2/3 of the American population are suffering from adrenal fatigue. These are modern ailments associated with our lifestyle with so much activity and so little time for rejuvenation and recuperation. It is also a result of our poor food supply, toxic environment, difficult relationships and not enough time for creative pursuits. These clients invariably have closed down or blocked third chakras. Opening the solar plexus up and rejuvenating the energy systems of the body brings energy levels back up to youthful levels. Many people look and feel younger just from this one remedy (in a very short time).

The Heart Portal represents your intuition and love

The heart portal is located in your heart center and fuels the heart, lungs, blood vessels, shoulders, ribs, breasts, diaphragm, and upper esophagus. Spiritual and emotional issues that can block energy in the heart are emotional expression; the capacity to fully express and resolve anger, hostility, joy, love, grief and forgiveness; the balance of giving and receiving and nurturing of self verses nurturing of others.

Physical maladies that occur with a weak or partially closed down heart portal are: heart attacks, hypertension, chest pain, congestive heart failure, asthma, allergies, lung cancer, pneumonia, upper back and shoulder problems, and breast cancer.

The nature of your heart is expansive appreciation and love for yourself (and others). When love for self is healthy and strong, generosity and love for others flow easily. The opposite of this is narcissism: self-obsession, selfishness and lack of connection or compassion to a benevolent divinity or awareness of others. It is basically a spirit that hasn't moved past infancy.

Your heart portal is located above the sternum, both front and back. It supports your heart, your circulatory system and your thymus gland, the key to your immune system.

Good colors for supporting the nature of love includes:

-**Red** provides affirmation to love and connection. Love is steady and constant, gentle yet the most powerful force on the planet. You create miracles with red as the power of love. When the heart chakra is in this purest form of red, the energy of the human resonates way beyond unconditional love and joy.

-**Pink for women** in the love chakra evokes nurturing female love. It will expand into her home family and immediate tribe. Pink for a man has him often perceived more as a girlfriend to women rather than a mate; he will be perceived as unable to provide and protect.

-**Green better for men than women**: For a man, green provides activation for his loving, divine self. His nature to protect and provide will rule his love interaction. For a woman, green often provides 'yang' or male energy providing balanced love.

-**Peach is** the color of love and happiness combined, a fun and nurturing version of healthy heart chakra.

-Orange in the heart chakra provides happiness in the love center. Here, love derives from self-actualization and self-affinity rather from another.

The heart portal can be broken but not missing; you can exist but not live without one.

While working with a two-year-old autistic child, Manuel, we could sense golden sparks were shooting into and out of his heart chakra. When I reached in to see what that was about, he was expressing his love and gratitude for having the parents he has. Despite his handicaps, his chakra told us what he couldn't express verbally.

The throat portal is energized by truth

The throat portal is found at the base of the neck, extending out from the hollow of the throat in front (clockwise spin) and in back (both clockwise and counter-clockwise spins). It represents your faith and higher communication. Here is where you discover your inner truth and use your voice to convey it to the world. Speaking half-truths and lies will block your throat and diminish your light.

Organs associated with the throat portal include the thyroid, trachea, neck vertebrae, throat, mouth, teeth, and gums. Spiritual and emotional issues that can block energy in the throat are the struggles between speaking versus listening, pushing forward versus waiting, and being willful versus compliant.

Physical maladies due to a weak or closed down throat portal are: bronchitis, hoarseness, chronic sore throats, mouth ulcers, gum difficulties, hypo or hyperthyroidism, chronic neck pain, laryngitis, swollen glands, and temporomandibular joint (tmj) problems.

It energizes communication, speech and language, whether oral or written. It is the sibling to the sacral portal in the area of communication, providing creativity related to the body while the throat provides creativity related to the mind.

Creativity flows from the inside out, providing a way for your inner thoughts and ideas to manifest to the outside world.

Good colors to support the nature of communication in order of their potency:

-Pink for women. Communication for a woman at its strongest is delivered from the space of nurturing and love. Pink provides for the amplification of love; it is the divine expression of female love. If a man would like to specifically lead women and match their energy to relay his communications to them, he would choose to have pink in the fifth chakra. A stronger choice for a man is green.

-Green for both men and women. For a man, green provides divine male love and healing in his communication chakra. For a woman, green provides balance in her communication. She will experience the yin-yang balance of her female nature to her assertive self.

-Orange: Communication fueled by happiness resonates as potent and something receivable.

-Blue is peaceful and still: good attributes for a peacemaker to embody. This facilitates change in, for example, a corporation or country.

One of the acts that can really harm your throat portal or chakra is that of not speaking the truth. Lying dims your light and when received by the person you're lying to, dims their light. Speak the truth without being brutal about it.

The Third Eye Portal fuels intuition.

Your third eye represents your intuition, intellect, visualization, imagination, and reasoning. Organs associated with it include the brain, eyes, ears, nose and pineal gland. Spiritual and emotional issues that can block energy there are struggles between clear and ambiguous perception, conservative and liberal morality, following rules and understanding that rules have exceptions, and repression and lack of inhibition. Physical dysfunctions that can occur from a blocked third eye are: brain tumors, stroke, neurological disturbances, blindness, deafness, tinnitus, Parkinson's disease, learning disabilities, and seizures. This portal allows the connection of our human spirit to our human body; it provides energy to our brain and center of head or golden temple of silence, which, it has been said, refers to the pineal gland or even the hypothalamus. The hypothalamus is the hormonal control center while the pineal gland allows us to go into a trance state, which allows us to access our subconscious directly.

Your third eye projects out from above the bridge of the nose in front and the back of the head. It provides access for inner vision and is female in nature, as it is inward in nature.

Good colors to support the nature of spirit-body union in order of their preference:

-**Blue/Indigo** as eternal peace is the highest expression of the brow center. Blues, especially in the deep rich colors, provide the stillness from which to observe life and choose wisely. In stillness, we come to know our true self as we discover our essential nature and transform/ascend to enlightenment. Meditation amplifies and quickens this spiritual progression. In the Siddha yoga tradition, there is a practice known as the blue pearl meditation. When a flash of blue appears in a thought process, it is said that this is the blue of truth and even blessing. This blue flash of insight means it is a truth should not be ignored.

-**Green** provides vitality in the sixth chakra.

-**Purple** provides a departure from the physical to a type of regality.

-**Yellow** provides the developmental energy wisdom. Fully embodied wisdom is royal blue.

-**Pink for both genders** provides essential knowledge related to love wisdom.

As you can see, the indigo color, which I see often on spiritually awake individuals, usually depicted for this portal is a good one but can also be other colors and still be healthy.

The Crown Portal: connection to the Divine.
Your crown portal is the connection of your spiritual nature and the Divine to your physical body. All organs in your body are associated with the crown portal or chakra. Spiritual and emotional issues that can block energy in the seventh portal include not understanding the nature of your existence and journey here on Earth. Your purpose may not always be clear but trusting that you have one will keep the channel clear. You do have influence on your life events but sometimes things just happen because of a circumstance. Maladies resulting from lack of connection with the Divine might be cerebral palsy, multiple sclerosis, ALS and any situation that serves as a wake up call.

Physically, your crown portal is positioned at the top of your head extends upwards straight rather than conically. People that are strongly connected and open will appear to have a bright column of gold or nearly white extending upward as far as you can see. You may also see yellow but it isn't nearly as powerful as gold. The receiving of energy through this portal provides energy for human growth in all aspects of your existence. It fuels brain function and body chemistry.

The color often depicted as purple is not a very good color for the crown; those with a purple crown feel and seem to be "invisible" to others, i.e., it is hard to get the attention of others. Other clairvoyant mediums have also verified this when I asked them.

Hand and Knee Portals

Hand portals, also known as nadis, are found on the palms of the hands and are vitally important for providing energy transmission or giving on the right hand and energy reception on the left. The left then is perfect for reading or understanding the information you are receiving while healing someone. With training, you can also use both hands for either function.

Knee portals, also nadis, are important to your loving yourself; they contain the metaphoric power of the ability to honor yourself.

Foot portals

Your feet provide an amazing map to the entire workings of the body. The bottoms of the feet provide the path to your soul understanding and allow you to channel healing Earth energy and allow you to ground yourself. Unlike the hands, the feet channels, located in the soft part of the foot towards the heel, are both receptive. Closed down foot portals may cause endless challenges because of the lack of grounding and connection. The portals are three inches in length, circular, and do not spin.

How to clear your portals

The first exercise that you'll need to practice is testing how open and clear your main portals or chakras are. You can use any random number system. I chose 0 to 100. Using my hand muscle test for yes and no, I start with, "Is it more than 50?" Then go up or down depending on my answer. So, I first test the root chakra and move up through to the crown. Very few people are open at all portals unless they've been in the regular practice of clearing themselves, either by listening to a clearing audio, doing work on themselves, or going to someone that can help them.

To clear them, I make a circular motion with my right hand as if I'm scooping out the blockages (see http://scientifichealer.com/book-bonus/). At the same time, I'm drawing healing energy (gold) down through my head and down my arm and using my right hand (and intentions) to help heal and clear anything in the way, allowing the energy flow in and out of the portals. If these are not cleared to allow easy flow of energy, whatever healing that might be done afterwards is less likely to last. In fact, reversion to the previous condition often occurs. A sudden miraculous healing of a condition is much like winning money in the lottery. If behaviors are not changed afterwards, the winner will be back in the same sorry situation as before much as lottery winners and their money situation within a year or two of winning big.

Likewise with a sudden healing. If the same forces are at play that brought you to the place of illness, it is unlikely that the newfound good health will last either. That's why the process in this book is comprehensive, not just about the healer bringing in healing energy to alter the current reality, but also actions that you can take to alter your own state. Health is a co-creation of healer and the one receiving the healing.

Once your ability grows and you become efficient, you can move through each portal, both major and minor, quickly and have them all cleared in minutes. To be sure, muscle test the numbers to make sure each opening is operating at 100 % capacity.

Reading:
Eban Alexander's encounter with the afterlife in "Proof of Heaven" http://scientifichealer.com/proof-of-heaven

Alex and Keith Malarkey's "The Boy Who Came Back From Heaven". http://scientifichealer.com/boy-who-came-back-heaven

What is your body field?

In an earlier chapter, I mentioned Dr. H.S. Burr, who measured energy fields around bodies (in the 1930s) and discovered that changes could be seen in this field long before illness manifested. Dr. Burr called this the L-field. It was not an idea that really took hold in the medical community although he was a classically trained M.D. Kirlian photography was developed at about the same time and revealed similar results, but this time what was measured became visible.

It is speculated that our energy fields are created when the spirit enters the body much as our energy channels are. While technically true, it is actually connected to the physical body as once the physical body is no longer alive, like the channels, the field dissolves.

Your nerve impulses, your organs, in particular your heart, your brain, your blood running through your veins, and your muscles all produce their own fields. Your heart field is the strongest, up to 30 times stronger than your nervous system. It has been measured out to 15 to 20 feet (about 5 to 6 meters) from your body. The view of the body field is that it reaches about our arm span or about three feet away from the body. All our biological activity will create fields around you and can be sensed by a person that is familiar with what to look for. For me, it is usually a tickling in the palm of my hands but it comes to me visually from time to time. It does not look like most of the pictures in books and on the web, at least not to me.

The healthier and more vibrant you are, the brighter and stronger your body field or aura. Not only is the vitality of your body and mind important, it is also what you project out to the world. Unresolved emotions, baggage from old relationships or past lives, issues you've inherited in your DNA and even negative thoughts and emotions projected at you by others ends up dulling your field (and causes a decrease in your vitality). What the dulling of your field looks like is that people don't see the real you, instead they will see only parts of you and it may be parts you don't want them to see.

Your field layers have been often attributed to various functions in other books, such as physical, emotional, etheric, etc. There are also assigned colors to the layers. However, those that see our fields note that we emit colors that correspond to our health and emotional state and this can vary even from moment to moment. Other psychic aura readers report events in your current and past lives as well as residue from interactions of others are stored there. So, the aura, your field, is a reflection of what is happening energetically in the body. In my experience, the latter explanation jives closely with what happens when I help clear the field of their negative energetic influences.

As soon as your field is cleared, not only can you see out more clearly, more people can see you clearly and see the real you. The negative influences cease to cause you to move off the tracks and goals you set for yourself. Life just becomes smoother and effortless.

Many of the illustrations of fields aren't how I've seen them. Your field is not just an even corona around your body but is more like a big teardrop where a column of energy goes up from the head (which may be an expression of the crown portal/channel). The field is complex, depending on the energy of the person or animal. Because of the added energy about the head, this may also be an expression of what is depicted as halos in saint icons and drawings. When a healer is fully lit, a haloed person is what you would expect to see if you are sensitive to seeing it.

There are many that will focus on mainly clearing your fields out. Using the Diamond Method protocols, a field clearing is just a small part of the process. Your field is a reflection of what is occurring within your body, mind, emotions, and spirit. Working from the inside out yields rapid results and appears more effective than just focusing on one aspect of the spiritual body.

For example, in working with some clients, I can feel a resistance around their body. If it's pulled out like a weed from the garden, it facilitates energy flow and makes some immediate problems disappear. Often the issue returns without the inner work.

Larry is one such example. He was urged to call me by a mutual friend. He wasn't sure who I was and what I did exactly but was suffering a bad headache from a chronic condition. When I got on the phone with him, I asked him if it was okay if I helped him with his headache. He agreed. As I'm asking him questions, not necessarily on his headache, but more about who he is and what he was doing at the moment.

As I reached into his field, I could feel something crackle, it felt like that static cling you get when the air is very dry. I yanked out the resistance and it felt like a weed was pulled loose. I threw it down a grounding cord (symbolically). As soon as it was out, Larry remarked, "I don't know what you just did but my headache just disappeared!" I finished out the session with the usual closing, which tells the body, literally: this is new programming; the old programming is obsolete. Larry had headache recurrences a couple of months later because he didn't "believe in" what I did for him although he experienced it and refused to change any life habits that could have helped.

Isn't my halo related to my aura?

There are some spiritual people that insist it is a different structure. It is difficult to tell because upon seeing a body field, as just mentioned, a halo like structure accompanies it above the head. The brighter someone becomes, the larger the halo appears as the field intensifies.

The stronger your field, the easier it is for you to interact with others at an unspoken level. Most people are "telepathic" in one form or another, especially if they are siblings or partners that are on the same wavelength. The stronger your field, the easier it is for you to draw in energy from your environment, good or bad. For healing yourself and others, it is possible to draw energy in from above through your crown, the back of your head, even through all your portals and through the entire surface of the skin. In part of the clearing process that is mentioned in the guided meditations, drawing the energy down from someplace that you love and makes you happy and running it along all your energy channels or meridians will clear up blockages and energize you. Your mind's intent is most important here: these concepts don't have to be real, just symbolic as your subconscious works symbolically.

Sometimes when I draw down large amounts of energy, my body will feel very lit up and even tremble a bit. When I've experienced this, those miraculous overnight healings have occurred: When Diane came to me with a large tumor in her back, basically at the 11th hour, she did not expect a miracle. She actually came to support her mother, Sarah, who was not doing very well with failing kidneys. Sarah had lost a lot of weight, looked haggard and drawn even though she was still only in her fifties. Diane also wasn't doing well, a 32-year-old mother of two was in chronic pain with back issues. Diane mentioned during her visit to my office that she was going to go through back surgery where her spinal sack was to be opened to remove a tumor in two days hence. This involved breaking the vertebrae open in that area.

Tears welled up in my eyes because I knew this procedure well. My mother had undergone it in 1971, after which she has been compromised and is now no longer ambulatory from over 40 years of spinal nerve deterioration. I knew that Sarah could be facing the rest of her life in a wheelchair or worse. My prayer was, "please don't let this young women with small children suffer like that." As I channeled the energy through me into her, my entire body trembled and I had goose bumps from head to toe, as I imagined the atoms and molecules in her back rearranging to form a perfect back exactly like the energetic blueprint she was born with. I thought I was a little crazy at that point but I went with it.

I kept my channels open for the entire next day and restructured Diane's back in my mind, using the concepts of quantum physics that I studied and even taught for the last 40 years. By the next evening, I had the image as clearly in my mind as if I were looking at a picture that her back was healthy, the tumor had disappeared. I sent her a message that she should ask that her back be re-imaged in the morning before the surgeon opened her up.

Indeed, the surgeon could not find any evidence of the tumor the next morning. She didn't need surgery. This was baffling to the doctors as the tumor had been seen in her back x-rays 3 times in the prior weeks. As a side note, Sarah now looks younger, radiant and healthier. Her kidneys are slow to regenerate, but she looks balanced and happy now.

Whether your halo is a separate structure or not, it's brightness or size is directly correlated with your clarity, which is directly correlated with how much healing energy you can draw down and direct.

Simple ways to clear your body field

Since the field is an energetic structure, it responds to the same kinds of things that anything electromagnetic would respond to such as grounding, using something magnetic, and filtering. Some like to use vacuums of one sort or another. I personally prefer grounding and magnets. Again, these are all symbolic forms of intent and since the mind is extremely powerful, the desired outcome usually results. A number of well-known top leaders use some sort of clearing daily. Robert Allen of "Nothing Down" and "Multiple Streams of Income" fame uses what he calls a squeegee. He brings an imaginary squeegee down through his body picking up all that doesn't belong there. I use an imaginary rose that has magnetic abilities and sweep it around the outside of my body, picking up the detritus that doesn't belong there, tossing it down a grounding cord when I'm done. Other healers might use a spiritual vacuum.

My brief guided meditation guides you through a process that will help you help yourself clearing out your channels, fields, adrenal glands (helpful for the highly stressed), sexual organs (which are also often ill), and bring you to a nice calm state. There are several that have been custom written for clients that needed extra help for their issues with great success. To see the current list, go to http://scientifichealer.com/audios/. The parasympathetic or healing state is the desired outcome without all the stressful energies that you usually carry around inside your body and fields.

Your spiritual timeline influences your present.

After your spiritual body is realigned and the channels and fields cleared, the first question that needs to be asked is whether your spiritual timeline is affecting your current situation. Your spiritual timeline is the ascension path from the time you first existed to now, and into the future. The model I use here is that we've lived before and are reincarnated several times. In each life, we experience new lessons that our soul wants to learn to ascend along a path to a higher level of existence or consciousness.

We keep experiencing the same lessons from lifetime to lifetime until we learn them, much like we do in a single lifetime. Thus, we carry an energy around certain issues, such as a lung problem for example. You may have had tuberculosis or pneumonia in other lives and now it expresses itself as asthma. When someone presents with a malady now, I always check to see if that energetic expressed itself along the spiritual timeline.

As I've mentioned, if you don't subscribe to prior lifetimes, then look at it as a working model that seems to dissipate the energy of issues affecting you now. It could be something else entirely, such as you inheriting this energetic from your ancestors. For now, the past life model works.

The model is that the energies from up to ten past lives can affect your present. If the origin of the energy is further back, it will be reflected in one of the last ten. Before that, the energy has already dissipated. I have read that some people will find an issue that originated 30 or 40 past lives ago and removing that influence will help the present. If the echo of this energy in the subsequent lives is not removed, it may still be an influence. However, not removing the energy from that long ago life but clearing the nearest ten lives WILL clear your current timeline from the influence.

An example of energetic influence could be that you always have a shoulder pain for which no doctor has found a biological cause. This could be due to an injury that was sustained in a previous life and the energetic echo is present in the current life. Once this is dissipated and the balance of the energetic issues resolved, the pain disappears. Another example might be an allergic reaction to a particular food. It may be that you got ill from eating tainted food in one lifetime; you may have even died from it. This energetic echo will carry forward in some but not all lives. Clearing this as well as other biological influences regarding this particular allergy will help alleviate the reaction to that particular food if not completely eliminate the allergic reaction.

While this removes the energetic influence of an allergy and will even seem to dissipate the allergy, before eating any particular food that you've reacted to in the past, you need to check with your doctor. The influence may be gone but you may still have other problems. Everything needs to be verified and tested.

Typical issues that have been removed are those overweight, diabetes, anger, depression, chronic pain with no biological root, anxiety, dementia, asthma, etc. While many people ask what exactly was the incident that imprinted the energy onto you such that it carried forth into the present life, I have not found it instructive or helpful for most people to dig into those reasons or events as often they are unpleasant memories and it just dredges them up over and over. Instead, it is just easier to remove the energetic influence without digging further.

To begin the process of clearing old influences, first determine which lives carry the energetic influence of a particular issue, beginning with the present and moving backwards to about 12 lives ago. Then use an energy clearing technique to pull that influence off the timeline. When I am clearing, I use a scooping motion and feel where it influenced the body as I work forward from the most distant time to the present. Often, this process reveals something important happening in the current life.

Debbie, a client with long standing back pain, came to me for some relief. As I was clearing off the influences, I felt a tugging in my legs and said it felt like they were different lengths. She assured me they were and she had never revealed that to anyone. I replied, that getting help for length issue, such as insoles in her shoes or chiropractic help, would be helpful in taming the pain. She did walk away from our sessions feeling free of the pain for the first time in many years after this clearing.

In a recent comparative study on those suffering chronic back pain to those not, there were the same structural anomalies in both sets of people, meaning that pain was not caused by the structural issue as much as an emotional/spiritual issue. This likely also speaks to those that have undergone back surgery for those same structural anomalies. For many, the surgery provides no relief.

Reading:
Power vs. Force, Dr. David Hawkins, for a clear discussion on Kinesiology and connection with the truth. http://scientifichealer.com/power-vs-force

All testing is via kinesiology or muscle testing, but has been verified with instruments when possible.

photo by Ozan, 2007

6. Your brain really does rule your entire being

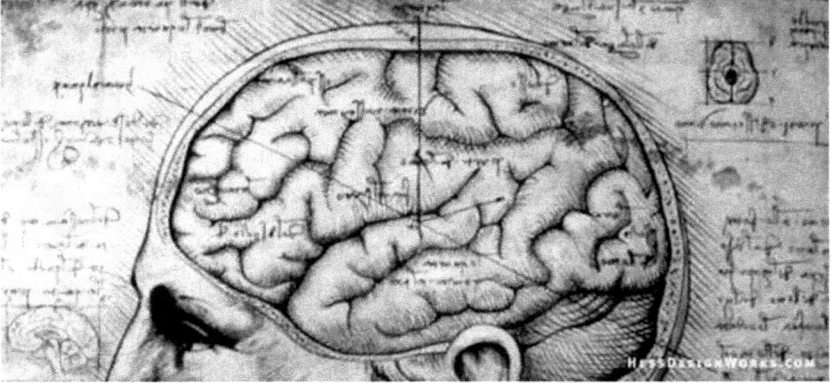

*"You must learn to let go. Release the stress.
You were never in control anyway."*
Steve Maraboli

The incredible evolution of man's brain

The number one fear that people have as they age is losing their identity and memory. This in itself is very stressful. The more fears you pile on yourself, the worse your life experience or perceptions of your experience will be. This is so unnecessary. There are a number of actions you can take to completely avoid brain decline with age. You can read in a number of books and plans that tell you to nourish yourself right, get plenty of rest, don't drink excessive alcohol or eat sugar, exercise your thinking, learning and analytical muscle, and exercise your body. Interestingly enough, one of the indicators of brain health in later years is muscle mass. If you maintain your muscles by maintaining an exercise program, your brain has a better chance of being healthy, vibrant and functioning until an advanced age. In this chapter, you'll discover that there are a few other things that will help you energetically which support those activities.

With this energetic support, you can overcome brain trauma as in George's unexpected recovery as well as reverse dementia, as you'll read about in Vanessa's remarkable case. These dramatic recoveries are not outliers, as we say in the lab, these are the norm. The outlier is the person who doesn't recover, where the cause lies in one of two directions. The first is the cooperation of the individual in supporting his or her own recovery and the second is stopping the work too soon. One or two sessions aren't going to reverse a traumatic injury or a lifetime of inertia. In George's case, it was several sessions over a three week period and in Vanessa's, it was an ongoing 4 month effort, weekly for the first month and then half sessions biweekly for three months to give you context. In learning the simple energetic principles you can do on your own, recovery is accelerated and made permanent.

Your Brain Rules

Your complex human brain really rules the body. If it is not in great health, your memory function declines with age, you may not be thinking as clearly as you might be (which can affect your relationships and income as well as your health), you may be in greater pain and you may not heal as quickly as you could. Your brain controls all glandular activity, which regulates many of the important functions of your body: your adrenal glands, pancreas, male and female organs, thyroid, and thymus. These systems are controlled by the hypothalamus and pituitary, which are both found in your brain.

Your healthy brain will also speed healing of pain, bruises and skin breaks, internal problems that cause limping, imbalance, lack of energy, etc. One of the things that was noticed early on in healings is that if your body chemistry was toxic, your brain would not sustain its health long term. One of the first parameters to look at is blood serum toxicity, such as, looking what toxins are in your food supply and environment.

Cognitive decline

One of the more common causes of cognitive decline is consumption of excessive alcohol and its sister molecule, sugar. It is well known that alcohol kills neurons and inhibits transmission of nerve and brain signals. So does lack of sleep, lack of exercise and poor nutrition. Further problems include the latest craze of excessive cholesterol control. A great proportion of our brains consist of cholesterol. The decrease of egg consumption along with an increase of cholesterol reducing drugs coincides with an increase in cognitive impairment amongst adults in their seventies and eighties and beyond. Improper nutrition limits the supply of the building blocks for neurotransmitters such as serotonin (tryptophan). Without neurotransmitters, our brains (and nervous system) cannot function as they are meant to.

There have been a few fascinating studies on cognitive decline including one memorable one involving a long term study of nuns and their brain function in order to understand the development of Alzheimer's, a form of dementia. Dr. DA Snowden started this study in 1986 and it still continues today, with many publications on their findings.

The nuns were asked to keep a journal of their daily activities and later, when they aged and died, a brain autopsy might reveal differences in which brains were functionally well at death and which weren't. Some of the very fascinating results of this study include: a) language mastery and complexity of thought was one of the best determinants of retained mental acuity, b) autopsies revealed little visual difference between healthy brains and brains that were compromised in function, and c) the initial stages of cognitive decline happened long before a crisis in symptoms appeared as the daily journaling revealed.

More information on brain function is coming to light: For example, your history of head injuries has a lot to do with decline of function later in life. Even small head traumas as a child may be affecting the function of the brain now. If, during your more active years of sports, say in high school or college, you participated in contact sports such as football, soccer or basketball, you more than likely sustained a number of minor if not major head traumas that have suppressed brain activities in the location of the traumas (or the opposite side of the head).

The body, especially head, retains the history of those traumas. Modern brain scans point this out very clearly. When injuries occur on a constant and sustained basis such as in contact sports, a declining ability to make good decisions, to think clearly, and to be pain free may be the result.

In all cases of declining brain function, improvement may be found via the Diamond Method protocols. In the case of Vanessa, an attractive 73-year-old former model, she had lost her ability to even remember what she did in the last half an hour, including eating, reading, watching TV, or interacting with her family. In other words, her dementia was quite advanced. Her husband was lonely and wanted his wonderful, vibrant, sassy, fun, and beautiful wife back. He also feared losing her soon because she also had a fairly large cancerous tumor in her breast.

The work proceeded with my speaking only to her husband, as she did not remember much. I could hear her voice in the background and connected with her this way. During the first month of weekly brain healing (each part of the brain as well as the brain organs are treated separately), she started having more interactive conversations and remembering her day better.

During the subsequent three months of biweekly checkups and tune-ups, her memory and abilities improved. She is now vibrant, active and remembers her week not just her day well. She is waking up earlier, has more energy, and enjoying outings more. As a side benefit, her cancerous tumor shrunk to a quarter of its size. It isn't just the brain that needs taking care of, but it is one of the main predictors of overall health and vibrancy at any age. Let's see what you need to know regarding brain function and healing.

Vanessa is a habitual heavy drinker of alcohol and despite this, she's had nearly a year of feeling like her old self. And without her knowing who I was and what I was doing to help her get healthy. This put to rest in my mind the possibility that a placebo effect was at work.

In the Diamond Method, there are five major key brain components that are rejuvenated separately:

1. The limbic brain: In many so-called primitive life forms, there is

no "brain" per se. There is only a grouping of neurons along the spinal cord that allow parts of the body to react as needed. As life became more complex, the brain followed suit. No matter how simple the organism, all vertebrate life forms on Earth have a primitive inner cortex called the limbic brain. This brain regulates many of the autonomic systems and supports the formation of memories and associated emotions and is the seat of the subconscious. The limbic brain is actually a collection of different brain structures with different functions, including the hippocampus, the amygdala, and the hypothalamus, which is the master controller for the glands and hormonal systems in your body. This is also called the primitive brain or lizard brain in English (in other countries, it might be called the crocodile brain).

The limbic brain is where your fight or flight response starts when an alarm of some sort startles you, whether it's a phone, fire alarm, siren or in ancient times, the proverbial saber tooth tiger. Your limbic brain signals the adrenal glands to fire off its hormones. The subsequent flood of adrenal hormones, including cortisol, adrenaline and aldosterone, send your nervous system into the sympathetic state, the state of high alert. In this state, you are not able to heal. In fact, it is a time when your body is using its resources rather than replenishing them. As you've already read, you will prematurely age and worse, get ill if you are too often in this state. Calming and soothing activities are important. The next chapter on stress will give you lots of clues and information on how to lower your stress levels naturally, without tranquilizers.

2. <u>The emotional brain</u>: The second part of the brain that's important for healing is the part of the limbic brain that controls emotions. Before you have thoughts, you have emotions. It is from this place that the subconscious operates. It is the real controller of many of our "conscious" actions. The subconscious thinks symbolically, which is why the use of symbols for healing works so well. For example, a rose is the symbol of love and purity and an imaginary grounding cord sent to the center of the earth symbolizes a lightning rod sending the excess energy away to protect us from harm. The subconscious isn't able to interpret certain language patterns. For example, it can't hear the word "not". So if you tell yourself, "I will not do that." The subconscious hears "do that". That's why telling a child to not do something usually prompts them to go ahead and do

it. Instead, commands need to be put in positive terms, as well as affirmations. Language will be covered in a later section.

In order for you to function in a family or societal group, to learn, to react appropriately in situations, your emotional to mental connection needs to be intact. As mentioned before, when you first encounter a situation, your first reaction is emotional. Thoughts are then formed from this emotion based on past history, emotional sensitivity to the situation, and inherited traits. Without this connection, we cannot react in a way that would benefit us.

An example of the inability to react properly is how an autistic person interacts socially. If someone approaches Don, an autistic man, while smiling, Don might just look at him without responding in any way. He doesn't realize that he is being recognized or approached in a friendly manner unless he was taught to react like that because it is what you're supposed to do. Don's emotions are not connected to his thoughts in the same way. Building that connection can help Don and it often does. Don normally responds to questions monosyllabically. Once the connections between his emotional and mental bodies are established, Don can now converse with longer sentences and smile in response when being approached.

3,4, and 5. The neocortex in three parts: The last parts of the brain that are important for healing separately surround the limbic brain and emotional center: the neocortex. The neocortex is divided into several lobes. For energy healing, only three basic dividing blocks seem to be important: the left and right neocortex each and the frontal lobes. The neocortex is involved with higher functions such as sensory perception, generation of motor commands, spatial reasoning, conscious thought and language.

The right neocortex controls the left side of the body and is the center for creative ideas and thoughts. The left neocortex controls the right side of the body and has a logical center important for analytical problem solving. The frontal lobes have an intuitive center; they control decision-making and are the origin of out of the box thinking and ideas. It's these areas that are often affected by head traumas while the inner brain organs are affected by lack of care in diet, self-care, and environment. The left and right neocortices contain the temporal lobes, which are involved in memory, language interpretation, and sensory input. Further functions found in the neocortices include speech, reasoning, emotions, learning, and fine control of movement.

There are four other brain centers that are handled separately: the hypothalamus, the master controller of the body and hormones; the pituitary, the second in command for hormones; the pineal gland, the melatonin producer important for sleep and meditation/relaxation; and the visual cortex found in the rear neocortex.

To what extent can brain trauma be repaired?

The extent to which brain trauma can be repaired by the Diamond Method protocol has not yet been fully tested. As you read early in this book, one of the biggest tests came in 2013 when a childhood acquaintance, George, was brought to the hospital after a truck had thrown him off his bicycle causing massive head injury and several broken bones. The doctors had declared him a lost cause; he would never recover and probably die in the following week or two.

Upon his recovery, the staggering realization is that we have enormous control of our future and we can choose which path our lives will take. A good brain healing basically changes your trajectory through life and profoundly so.

To describe at this point exactly what measures are taken to heal the brain fully is premature because so much is involved that has not yet been covered. The basic steps are to first do a methodical diagnostic reading, which dictates which process to begin first then go through the balance step by step. The path is not clear at the outset because as each process is completed, the next step to take is revealed. By using this methodical approach, it allows anyone to be able to go through the entire protocol without the benefit of special intuitive gifts.

You've already learned about the beginning of the process in the previous chapter, which includes making sure the spirit is in the body. Next, the body's energy channels and fields are cleared of negativity and blocks, which can be done by yourself using the simple meditation audios available through the links in this book. Further steps in the process will be covered in subsequent chapters. This chapter now covers the effective reprogramming of your brain, which in turn help you make better choices and promotes more healing.

Ways to keep brain health going for a long time

There have been a number of books and studies on this topic, as Alzheimer's and dementia are looming large these days. Families are having fewer children forcing the average age of our population up. There are several points that all the studies agree upon: healthy food, low alcohol and sugar consumption, exercise, sleep, low exposure to toxins whether work or home, no recreational drug use, keep brain injuries to a minimum (in other words, contact sports are dangerous to the brain), drink plenty of fluids, healthy fat intake, and eating your veggies. These are the obvious healthy brain activities.

Secondary activities include keeping the thinking muscle active such as learning new subjects, undertaking new activities, and solving puzzles to lay down new neural pathways as well as keep the old ones in use. Muscle building exercise is particularly important as healthy muscle retention as you age is indicative of brain health. Last, reducing negative emotions, especially fears and anxieties, keep neural patterns healthy and the brain plump and juicy. You'll read about emotions later in this chapter.

The words you use not only reflect how you think, it also affects your thinking.

Your brain is an amazing "computer", it can make almost any reality appear. Given this incredible power of creation, language is extremely important. How you speak to yourself is really the difference between being overtired/stressed and going through life with ease and grace. A perfect example of effectiveness of words is how often the future is determined by what an authority figure may have said to you.

For example, doctor's proclamations and declarations are often self-fulfilling prophesies. If you've been told you might have two, maybe three months to live, tops, due to a condition, usually the body complies. This is a poor but common practice amongst medical professionals.

Some people complain that they'd rather know so they can take care of unfinished business. Rather than procrastinate until it is too late, it would be better to enjoy each day with all the loose ends taken care of. Such actions could include making up to people you may have had a disagreement with, paying your bills on time, and making sure you have a will for your heirs.

Instead of predicting how much time you have left, wouldn't it be better to focus on returning your body to a healthy state given the information you find in this book and others like it? The conventional tactic of prescribing medications and surgery isn't enough. With the amazing recoveries I've seen from hundreds of clients, it looks as if you can heal from virtually anything. The possibilities are really limitless. It is only limited by what you can see for yourself and how you speak to yourself.

Having upbeat and positive thoughts also improve brain function dramatically, according to brain scans.

Successful people have a common set of thoughts.

They don't give up the first time they trip. They always get right back up and keep going. Things can look pretty bleak if an outsider viewed the process, but the successful people keep going. They use a process which includes setting goals, finding their motivation, keeping their language positive, and planning, planning, planning. Then the plan is worked. If you get up every morning and write down a list or schedule (and this only takes a few minutes at most), you will get a lot more done, for example.

The subconscious is symbolic and powerful

It preserves and runs the body on old programming. Unless you make a conscious effort to reprogram it, old programs will continue to run and even sabotage your life. Therefore, the strategies below accelerate the reprogramming process.

The subconscious is literal. It doesn't understand irony, it doesn't take in certain words or concepts, such as negatives. Such as, if you say to yourself, "don't get fat." Your mind hears "do get fat." The subconscious operates on instinct and habit. You can use repetition, authority and emotion to reprogram it. These include affirmations.

Memories of situations with negative emotions get repressed yet the emotions and beliefs will still control your actions. The subconscious mind works with symbols and metaphors. Symbols and rituals help in reprogramming. Several of the exercises that we do use certain universal symbols to effectively process negative thought patterns, behaviors, and baggage from negative relationships out of the body. For example, for most of the rose is a symbol of love and purity and can be used as such to help remove negative energy or evil.

The subconscious has the psyche of a sensitive five year old; it takes everything personally. It takes the path of the least resistance, which usually means the more negative path of the offered choices. You need to engage your conscious mind to make positive changes in your life. Your subconscious has a need to be moral, meaning that it supports your moving towards a higher level in your spiritual journey. And last, it doesn't have a sense of time. Everything it feels is now. There is no past and there is no future. Therefore, any and all affirmations need to be spoken in the present tense.

Step one: Focus on the positive and gratitude

There is something magical about focusing on gratitude. Gratitude forces you to think about everything that is right with your life, the parts you love, the people you love and the good things you enjoy having. The way the mind works is that when it focuses on the positive it will bring more of that into reality. If you look at the house you live in as a good thing, no matter how modest, you will enjoy having it and you'll take care of it and make sure it always looks good. The better you make it, the more you will like it and the more valuable it becomes.

You could do the same with your relationships, your job and your health. For example, let's say your job is not ideal. For most, a job that is not ideal is a source of stress.

But let's say that you have a coworker you enjoy, you like living in the city you're in and you have some tasks you enjoy. If you focus your gratitude on having a job that helps pay your bills, on having a coworker you enjoy or tasks you might enjoy or even being able to live in a city you want to stay in, you'll find that more parts of that job will improve and that you might be doing so much better at getting tasks done that your bosses take notice.

No one likes a grumbling or complaining employee. Employees are expensive risks and when someone starts stirring the negativity pot, it spreads to other employees and causes productivity to go down. When there's a positive employee that is grateful for the chance to work and have a good job, the positivity spreads, and you'll find favor with those bosses. This contributes to improving your work situation.

Let's look at what happened with Leann. She started with an oil company shortly after completing graduate school. She had enjoyed research and presenting new results to other scientists. The oil company job was lucrative but when she arrived, she was placed in a lab that was months behind in their work, had a huge inventory of old samples that were poorly documented, and much of the work that it did for other parts of the company was not on record. It felt like drudgery after grad school.

Leann started with gratitude: she was thankful she had a good paying job, great coworkers, and liked living in her city. She put an action plan in place to get her lab caught up, the completed work on record by recruiting her staff to help generate reports of every analysis/transaction taking place within the lab, and worked with her senior lab tech to document the piles of old samples. As her bosses took notice, they offered her large raises and a bigger budget for her lab. She was able to buy instruments to start doing more original research, which led to more autonomy, more salary and more recognition. After a short time, her job transformed from drudgery to totally satisfying and enjoyable.

Exercise: Make a gratitude list of at least three things every morning. Recite them out loud.

Step two: Focus on the positive: Affirmations

Give the solution, not the problem, the energy. "I don't want to be fat", "I don't want to be poor", "I don't want to be sick", "I don't want to give up my lifestyle" and "I don't want to have cancer" are poorly stated affirmations. They give the problem the energy, rather than the solution. As mentioned, your subconscious doesn't pay attention to the negative words, it hears: I want to be fat, I want to be poor, I want to be sick and I want cancer. If it is reframed as a positive statement, your subconscious will help propel you towards your goals. Even better, state it in the present. I am lean (better to state the exact weight). I am healthy. I am rich (better to state the exact amount of money or goods that it will take to feel rich). All my cells are healthy. I am strong (better to state how much you can now lift). I have great relationships. I live in the best house (better to state exactly what that looks like to you).

Great affirmations are stated in the present tense as if were already true. They need to be believable. For example, if you are earning two thousand dollars a month, writing an affirmation that $100,000 appears in my bank account every month won't ring true and your conscious gate keeper won't allow that through. It's better if it is an achievable goal in your mind. It would be better to use eight or ten thousand instead.

Great affirmations do not state how you are going to achieve the goal, only that it is reached. Even saying you are going to earn something implies work. It is better to say it as if it magically appears. I weigh 118 lbs is better than saying that you lost the fat by some process.

Write affirmations and goals on cards and carry them around. During any idle moment, read them out loud. Say them at least once if not twice a day.

Step three: Find your emotional reason for succeeding.

Without having a strong emotional motivation, it is easy to fall back into old bad habits: your subconscious will have no reason for changing. For example, it could be you want to live long enough to see your children graduate from school. Or you must do it or you will have a heart attack in 6 months (according to your doctor). A lot of people starting in their late 50s fear their mortality much more than younger people. It's frightening getting old and that fear will get us motivated.   Many of my clients are in that over 50 age bracket: they have been doing what they thought were the right things but they still ended up somehow ill, tired, or unable to cope. They are motivated to feel like they did in their 20s again and be productive and healthy for a lot longer. It's available to all of you.

Exercise: think about your biggest current goals and see if you can attach a big emotional reason to achieve that goal. It has to be big, deep and important. It can even be an expensive pervasive problem that needs urgent attending to.

Step four: Set clear goals.

There is a big difference between knowing what to do and doing what you know. Writing out your goals is very important. Many people use 3x5 index cards and carry them in their pockets to remind them.

Set very specific goals: Setting specific goals instead of vague ones are one of the biggest keys to success. For example, if your goal is to lose some weight to help lower your cholesterol, then put down the specific number of pounds. Or perhaps your goal is to find your soul mate, earn a specific amount of money by a certain time or live in a specific dream house by a certain date. Writing these as positive affirmations is the most powerful: "I weigh xxx lbs." "I live in a 2000 sf house with an ocean view in Southern California." "20 thousand dollars flows into my bank account every month."

Put a time limit on your goal – For example, use a two month time limit. If today is December 1st, for example, write "Today is Feb 1st and I weigh xxxx lbs."

Set big long term and overall goals. Best is if you have goals for every time period: one year goals, 3 month goals, one month goals, weekly goals and daily goals. A daily goal could be, for example, to drink two liters of water and take a 30 min walk. This would be an excellent start into a new healthy program.

Step five: Use visualization.

Create a vision board for everything you want to manifest. Get out an old lean or healthy picture of yourself and put it on the frig, your computer, your door, and a copy in your pocket. If you were never lean, borrow someone else's lean body and photoshop your face onto it. You can look, do, have, or be like that again, no matter what anyone says. A good place to go is Shape, Health, or Men's Health magazine to get pictures of healthy people to help visualize how you will look as a lean, healthy person. Imagine your dream house, your dream man or woman, or your dream vacation. Hang your vision board in a prominent place to keep reminding you of what you are working towards.

Step six: Plan ahead and be prepared for contingencies

Success doesn't just happen, it requires planning. Include anything that could go wrong and get you off your path so you have no excuse. When you go to the gym, put down your workout ahead of time and then just follow the plan. When you go shopping, make a list of what you need and then go get it. Why not plan out your meals (sample meal plans are given later), decide what you need to shop for, and decide at least a day or two in advance what those meals will look like and when. Use an alarm or timer to remind yourself when you need to eat. Plan what your work strategy is, whether it is to call your new prospects, get that report done, or do your essential bookkeeping. This is important. Your life depends on it.

Once new habits are established, the planning becomes automatic and takes almost no time. If you are going on a trip, plan how and when you'll take a walk or exercise, where and how you will eat or find good food to eat. Cook protein in batches, then make smaller meals of them, which takes only a few minutes to make a quick salad, or stir fry some veggies with bits of the cooked chicken, steak or fish. When you go to work, pack meals the night before using the precooked chicken or hamburger along with whatever veggies. You should be able to prepare 4 out of the 5 small meals and snacks that you eat all day in about 15 minutes. This is considerably less time than it takes to run out at lunchtime to find a sandwich or find a fast food place, plus you're getting the healthy food you need.

There are always instances that make it difficult to stick to your plan. For eating and health, you might find parties difficult with too much drinking and the wrong food, for example. Offer to bring something that works for you because the usual fare isn't very healthy. Or you can eat a good meal ahead of time so you're not tempted by the unhealthy food. Once you're nourished and satisfied, unhealthy food is less attractive or tempting. If you're invited over for dinner and you don't know the people well, try bringing something in a pocket or bag that will replace some of the meal in case there is nothing you can eat. We've all been to enough events in our lives that we pretty much know what is going to happen. Always carry supplies with you to make sure you're not tempted. Once you are used to this, it works quite well and is discrete (don't make an issue of it and focus on the people instead of the food). If you look around, you might find other people doing the same thing.

For career related situations, it is always tempting to take too long at break, gossip, or waste time surfing on the Internet. That won't help you succeed and reach any goals. Instead set goals by making a list ahead of time of the three major tasks you wish to achieve today, set time limits on how long you'll spend at each and follow the plan.

Step seven: Reframe language.

One way to insure success is to reframe our normal language from focusing on the problems to focusing on the solutions. "Problems" become "challenges," "failure" becomes "feedback (or data)," "frustration" becomes "fascination," "should" becomes "must," "older" becomes "wiser," "an injury" becomes "an inconvenience." Use positive language, instead of saying "if I accomplish," say "when I accomplish." Describe your past as challenging rather than problematic or that you learned something or you grew wiser and stronger during the process you went through. Describe some undesirable trait as something that's in your past.

Beliefs are not facts. There are studies all over that can prove anything you want: eggs are good, eggs are bad, cigarettes are good, cigarettes are bad, margarine is good, margarine is bad. The end result is that we are getting more and more confusing information. Usually, common sense prevails. The facts are discoverable if you look and know how to interpret them. I hope you will learn some critical thinking from the pages of this book so you can read the studies for yourself and find the monkey wrench in the works if the study just plain doesn't make any sense.

Just because something doesn't work the first go around, means more research data is needed: Remember, Thomas Edison described his 1000 failures to make a light bulb before he succeeded: "I didn't fail, I just found more than 1000 ways it didn't work."

Last, you may have heard of the seven beliefs of highly successful people. It is based on their self-talk. Thomas Edison probably believed this too.

It's achievable.

I am able

I must achieve it

I deserve it

I want it

I expect it

I am willing to do what it takes.

Homework

Successful health, wealth and relationship management can be fit into any lifestyle. First and foremost, success requires motivation.

Write your motivation on a 3 x 5 card and carry it with you. Take it out often. Examples may be:

1: I now have a cholesterol level of 190 so I can live longer and improve quality of life

2: I now have perfect health so I can take better care of my children/wife/husband/company/parents or have more fun sailing, going to Hawaii, or seeing Europe.

3: I now have a blood pressure of 120/80 so I can get off drugs that are causing me unpleasant side effects (such as sexual dysfunction, joint pain, poor memory, muscle pain).

4: I now weigh 170, my ideal healthy weight, so I can look better, leaner, sexier, more desirable, or find my ideal mate.

5: I live in a 2000 sf house in San Diego overlooking the ocean.

6: My yearly income is $360,000.

The power of the subconscious is our strongest ally. We all deserve to be in good health so we can live our best lives.

Write very specific goals with time frames as in item 4. Set time limits. If you want to lower your cholesterol to a certain number, if you want to weigh less by a certain number, put a time limit on it.

"My cholesterol is 100 points lower than 30 days ago."

"I weigh 10 lbs less than 30 days ago."

"I live in an ocean view home."

"I am married to my ideal mate."

How your emotions affect your health and happiness

Like anything in our bodies, whether it is a thought, something physical such as nerves or glands, or an emotion, it has its own characteristic energy. With that characteristic energy, it has its own frequency. You'll hear the term "raise the frequency of the planet" often these days. You might wonder as I did what that meant. It actually means more people will be moving up the frequency ladder of emotions. You'll see later, that this means they are moving from an externally driven emotional life to an internally driven one.

The quality of your life, your health, your relationships and your wealth will tell you how you're doing emotionally. As soon as you change the emotions that are "vibrating" in our bodies, you alter who is around you and even your fate. Releasing the negative emotions drives your body back into the parasympathetic or healing state by calming your adrenal glands.

We tend to attract people (a) similar to us or (b) those that we need to learn from. We will repel those that don't want to deal with our emotions because basically, we are wearing them, no matter if we are positive or negative. You would think that positive people would attract everyone, but they don't. Haven't you ever heard the term "Pollyana" behavior as if it were derogatory or wrong? There is nothing wrong with finding the gift in whatever circumstance you're experiencing or have prevailed over.

All low vibrating emotions hurt us. The key to mental and physical health is spiritual and emotional health. You could ask, "why do we have those negative emotions if they're harmful to us?" The dark emotions such as fear, anger, and sorrow do bring our energies down because they consume us. They are actually meant to protect us and propel us to change. In reality, they are temporary and are not you. They do not reflect who you are, only who you are being at the moment. You can transcend actions and emotions and become the healthy being you were always meant to be.

We can store negative emotions almost anywhere in our body although they tend to be stored in certain glands, organs or systems. The event that stored this negative emotion could be something that occurred while a fetus, an infant, a child, or later. It could also have occurred in a past life. In addition, you can also inherit stored emotions from your parents or other relatives related to your parents that came before them.

The reason why this can occur so easily is that the frequency of that emotion resonates with certain parts of the body, glands, organs or anywhere else. While the negative emotion is resonating in a parent's body, it can be transmitted to the fetus. The stored emotions can be released by processing them, talking through them, or via the Diamond Method protocols.

The advantage of the Diamond Method over traditional methods is that you don't have to talk about the same things over and over again that caused you pain in the first place. You don't need to relive them, remember exactly what and why, and keep going back to that uncomfortable place again and again. In the case of my own difficult circumstances, retelling for the umpteenth time did not relieve the pain but just made me hurt all over and over again. I had learned the lessons I needed to, I wasn't going to go back to the old behavior that got me to that place. My releasing them via the Diamond Method allowed me to let everything go, be free of them and move on in grace and ease.

How emotions are trapped.

No one wants to feel low energy emotions, such as anger, fear or anxiety. You tend to bury them somewhere so you can move forward without acknowledging them. The subconscious stuffs them somewhere in your body to avoid feeling their discomfort. But these emotions are useful to us. Fear is to help us survive in dangerous situations. Anger is for us to realize when our boundaries have been crossed. And sorrow is to slow us down to accept a loss.

Most of us do not take the time to recuperate, to process them, and go back to nature and self-care. We try to keep going, keep functioning, and keep doing what we've always done. As these accumulate, the level of stress that is felt increases while our adrenal glands get beaten up and over used until they fail.

The trapping of an emotion starts when you first encounter something; your first reaction is an emotion, then the thoughts follow. You start thinking of the reasons you've had that emotion and its intensity, filling in a full story. Later, if you've stored an emotion in your body, you'll be sensitized to it, meaning you'll be very quick to respond to anything that appears similar to the event that caused it in the first place. You can recognize when this happens, especially in other people, because their reaction to a situation seems out of proportion to the incident. In reality, you or the other person is reacting not just to the current incident but also to everything else in his/her life that caused that emotion to store itself in the body.

Many times, the emotions are trapped when we are very young and cannot process them out very well because we are incapable of the reasoning that it takes to work through them immediately. Sometimes the things our parents told got us stuck in the first place. It doesn't compute when someone that is supposed to love us and take care of us tells us that we are no good in some way, shape or form. Then the emotion gets trapped.

Many times in troubling relationships, whether it's a partner, parent, child, or other relationship, there's some sort of emotional charge. The source of the emotional charge is difficult to determine because it's buried deeply and masked by layers of incidents related to that emotion.

Let's look at what happened in the case of Susan and John: they go to dinner and Susan sends back a meal because it wasn't made the way she wanted (perhaps the steak was overcooked). John is furious and wants Susan to just eat the steak and stop being so nit-picky. In counseling, Susan complained that John got really angry that she sent her poorly prepared food back.

When John was asked why got angry, he says, "Susan is never satisfied. And her actions embarrass me." But why should sending poorly prepared food back get such a rise out of John? He'll make up almost any reason he can grasp at but he isn't aware of the real issue. He can't even imagine what it is.

John is sensitized to something in his wife's reaction that makes him feel inadequate because he placed the order for her. So he feels he is not providing for her well enough and she might desert him for it. He has a strong fear of abandonment buried beneath all the bluster.

When you step back, it seems like a stretch until you consider that he has a negative emotion, fear of abandonment vibrating somewhere in his body and it has sensitized him to feeling like a poor provider and worried he'll end up alone.

He feels stuck in a situation for which there seems to be no solution because the real issue isn't ever brought to light. Yes, this is a real story and it did happen just that way and those were the reasons.

The energy of emotions

Dr. David Hawkins muscle tested hundreds if not thousands of people to determine how energetic various emotions are. He set up a geometric scale from one to a thousand to classify a set of emotions. The classifications are based on whether having the emotion drives the person externally or internally, with a dividing line of 200. Below 200, a person is externally driven and as they move above 200, they become more internally driven.

An externally driven person cares about what others think of them and their actions, they worry about appearances, and are jealous of what other people have, for example. An internally driven person cares about his or her behavior because it matters to them and doesn't worry about what others think. For example, an internally driven artist would create outrageous original work because they are busy exploring new media and new ways of self-expression while an externally driven artist would worry if anyone would buy their art and if it is good enough.

The emotions below 200 in increasing value are shame, guilt, apathy, grief, fear, desire, anger, and pride while those 200 and above are courage, neutrality, willingness, acceptance, reason, love, joy and peace. Hawkins classified vibrations above 600 as enlightened, meaning we cease to have an ego and we are in the bliss state or pure consciousness, which is our core nature.

First, on any single day, we can have a range of emotions. We were made to have them: the negative emotions serve as protection and impetus for change. Any time we are in emotional pain, we seek to move out of it. So, your measurement on this scale can vary from day to day although we can be at a natural state when we are in "neutral" so to speak. The more stressed and over-whelmed we become, the lower we'll land on the scale. I worked with a powerful and amazing healer who had measured me anywhere from 400 to 600 on the Hawkins scale on any given day. Thus, some of the statements in Hawkins' book don't seem to jive with the observations of others.

There are a number of programs, classes and healing modalities based on moving up the scale. Anyone that has "point envy", that is wanting to be higher on the scale but isn't, is low on the scale and ambitious. Anyone that is higher on the scale doesn't really care because as an enlightened, loving or joyful person, you feel so good, you don't care where you land. I find this system a little stifling on the one hand because people feel boxed in and the book specifically states that one can only move up the scale about 15 points in a tough lifetime. Artificially raising the levels instead of learning life's lessons, according to the author, has repercussions, much as a slingshot, sending a person deeper into trouble. For example, drugs might send someone into that blissful state, thereafter causing him/her to become an addict and neglect his/her life.

The instructive part of the scale is that it shows the emotional frequency of vibrations, whether they are low or high energy. To picture how the frequencies can resonate somewhere in the body, imagine a piano or guitar string, once plucked, vibrates at a specific frequency. The heavier the string (the wrapped ones are heavier per unit length), the lower the frequency. Those strings can actually vibrate at several frequencies depending on how fast the wave is traveling up and down the string. It can vibrate at any frequency as long as the wave is multiples of the length of the string. These are called overtones and what make some music sound very beautiful. Our organs are much the same way. They can vibrate at a high frequency or a lower one. In this case, when it is low, the organ will feel heavy and sluggish.

Our organs vibrate with certain emotions and the types of emotions are determined by how they align along certain of the acupuncture meridians. You'll find anger emotions store easily in the liver and gall bladder, fear emotions in the kidneys and bladder, while sadness will store in the lungs and heart. You probably have heard the term "heartbroken" or that someone was so frightened, he/she wet his/her pants or that rising bile meant anger. These emotions resonate and reside in those organs.

Where emotions are trapped

Emotions can get trapped in our bodies in various places, not just those organs. Human emotions can be divided in four basic categories. The rest are nuances and mixtures of these, much as all colors we perceive are mixtures of three basic colors plus lightness/darkness. For example, pink is light red and brown is dark orange. These four basic emotions are fear, happiness, sadness, and anger. I find them easy to remember as mad, sad, glad, and fear.

Nuances of fear emotions are anxiety, dread, worry, insecurity, terror, and nervousness; of anger emotions are bitterness, guilt, hatred, resentment, and jealousy; and of sad emotions are grief, discouragement, sorrow, sadness, depression, heartache, and feeling forlorn. This is by no means an exhaustive list.

In working with my private clients, I've seen dramatic shifts happen when these trapped emotions are released. As I work with them, I can feel the warmth of higher vibrating energy rush into their organs and body.

In the case of Louise, after releasing years of pent up anger, her demeanor changed so much that people asked, "What happened to you? You're so happy, cheerful and energetic now." Her phone started ringing off the hook with clients and her income has taken a sharp upward turn. Another client, Lucy, was telling me that since working with me, especially on her emotions and feelings, her business has taken a sharp upward turn and that her income will increase 2 to 3 times more than before.

The reason income is affected is that income is based on relationships, whether you're selling your services, widgets, or work in an organization. Often being hired hinges on whether you fit in with the other employees, not your competence. Stored negative emotions are felt by others, even if you are acting pleasant, are polite, and you like people. Those negative emotions will emanate outwards and be felt even before you walk in the room.

In the protocols for checking the energy body, examining the body and energy field for stored emotions comes right after checking the spiritual body, both body fields and energy channels. If buried emotions are found, they are then replaced with healthy emotions and the emotional charge for similar situations gets grounded and released. The response is then more in balance, more control, and less volatility.

The relief may happen immediately or may take a few days for the body's energy systems to readjust to its new state of vibration. When the negative emotion has been drained, people report they feel a lot more powerful because they feel more in control.

Here's a recent situation for Joseph: Joseph felt cheated out of a sales commission even though he had helped bring the client to purchase the product. The client attended a workshop then bought a big-ticket item. Joseph also had a coworker that pushed his buttons and made him feel out of control. When Joseph brought up the commission, he would gripe and yell and no one gave him what he was really due. That coworker knew just what to say to drive Joseph crazy. Joseph didn't really understand why what they just said bothered him so much. And what's worse, Joseph felt they had the upper hand.

After working with Joseph, the negative emotion, anger over being cheated, was drained out of the liver; those hot reactions are no longer present. He was surprised that the next time he was shortchanged on his commission, he could calmly and clearly express what he wanted. Joseph was delighted that he was no longer out of control and barking back. Instead, his calm and logical reasoning with his coworker got him his requested commission and bonus. Now Joseph has power over these situations, not his coworker. He can now choose how he responds rather than responding with a knee-jerk reaction.

Where are the consequences of trapped low energy emotions?

As mentioned, our organs resonate with the frequency of low energy emotions. For example, fear emotions such as anxiety, dread, worry, insecurity, terror, and nervousness tend to get stored in the kidneys and bladder. They can also appear in the heart, lungs and stomach. Anger emotions such as bitterness, guilt, hatred, resentment, even jealousy tends to be stored in the liver and gall bladder. Sad emotions such as grief, discouragement, sorrow, sadness, depression, heartache, and feeling forlorn tend to be stored in the lungs and heart. If your field were to be measured as Dr. Burr did, it would read a lower field around those organs leading to problems.

A trapped negative emotion basically dims the light of the area in which it is trapped. It lowers the energy by dropping to a lower frequency. The basic rule of energetics is that energy is proportional to frequency. With lower frequency, that part of your body is not being fed properly; it doesn't have enough energy to repair itself, sustain itself, and be free of tumors, cancer, premature degeneration, calcification, and inflammation. Measurements of fields around bodies prior to illness show this to be clearly the case, that illness manifests itself in the energy fields long before it physically manifests.

For example, imagine a low energy emotion is lodged in your liver, some form of anger perhaps. Your liver resonates and vibrates at a lower level. This lower energy is not enough to keep it in perfect health so over the long haul, your liver will start to have problems, say non-alcoholic liver disease or even fail to regulate cholesterol properly. This can affect your entire health as the liver performs 17 major functions of your body, such as cleaning up toxins, regulating cholesterol, providing energy to the muscles, storing glycogen, etc.

When the anger is released from the liver, the light is restored. The light can then vibrate at the higher frequency, bringing energy and vitality back. The field around it will register stronger. Health to the liver can eventually be restored if not quickly.

In Louise's case, the woman with all that anger stored for over 40 years, her immune system had failed and she was unable to fight off illnesses. She was on a nearly constant prescription of antibiotics and a slew of other expensive medications. Her liver was borderline. Healing it alone physically would have been only a stopgap measure. It would soon be back to its sick self had the negative emotions stayed stuck inside. Releasing them was a huge step forward. Now for the first time, she is free of lung congestion and antibiotics.

In Lucy's case, her fears and frustrations warded off her potential valuable clients. For her, each client is worth tens of thousands of dollars to her bottom line and each loss meant having to go out and work in a day job she hated to put food on the table.

A clearing is not permanent; if you re-engage in the previous behaviors, you can be re-infected. The whole idea of having the emotion in the first place was to get you to change your behavior. Sometimes, the patterns are so familiar to you that they're easy to fall back into. It takes awareness of this to stay clear, that and positive actions so you don't fall back into old habits. That's where learning some basic clearing techniques for yourself is very important, either that or going back to a Scientific Healer to be cleared, grounded and healed of that issue and reinforce the original healing. It also takes changing your daily routines a bit, small readjustments, to show your psyche how much you care for yourself. This small shift can make all the difference.

Sometimes, people are very layered. There are other buried emotions that cause the same kind of reaction. If you remove a layer, another one rises to the surface. Removing more than three buried emotions at any one sitting isn't recommended, as the change can be too large, causing a healing crisis. So, letting it settle or adjust for a week or so, then removing another layer is helpful to smooth the adjustment period. Eventually we do get to the end or at least where it's only small adjustments, not massive ones.

You are never too old.

In my experience, age doesn't seem to matter. Removing the emotion from an organ or body part works just as effectively on someone in their 80s as it is from someone in their 20s. A younger person heals a little faster physically, but emotionally, older people are just as easy to adjust. Older people sometimes realize after the clearing of that emotion that there's a whole other way to be that they never experienced and they enjoy it.

The only requirement is to be ready and open to this kind of healing. Being willing to release all that was before and be ready to embrace what is to come.

Some people are fearful of an unknown future. Arnold was one such person. The first time I asked him if he wanted help with an issue, he said that he was all right. But he wasn't all right, because he struggles with the vestiges of a massive brain injury over 30 years ago caused by him being propelled through the windshield of the car he was a passenger in. It takes faith to trust in the process, letting go and let things happen as they are supposed to. No matter where you are in your path, you are in exactly the right place.

There are a number of things you can do to help maintain a healing, any healing. First, respect and honor your body. This gives your mind the signal that you value yourself and you deserve to be strong and healthy. Rest well, exercise, eat well, drink plenty of water, stay away from alcohol and over the counter drugs/recreational drugs, don't smoke, and lower your stress levels. Second, use positive language to describe yourself and those around you. Watch positive programming, listen to positive music, read positive uplifting books, and hang out with positive people. Positivity is contagious and you'll help propel yourself forward along your path to perfect health. Third, do simple energetic groundings and clearings. You could do this in under 15 minutes a day: listen to the brief clearing meditation found at http://diamondhealingmethod.com.

Telling your body that you really care, that you are valuable, puts you in a state of mind that you want to heal and stay well after that.

How to clear emotions.

Clearing emotions is done much the same way as clearing any excess energy in the body. It's done by grounding. After working with hundreds of clients, the minimum requirement is that the location and the emotion be identified. The source of the emotion isn't necessary although some clients really want to know what caused it in the first place. I try to supply as little information as possible so as to not stir the unpleasant memory so the client doesn't anchor the unpleasantness with being healed.

What you want to avoid is to bring up the hurtful or distasteful memory again. I have not found it to be cathartic. Some people will end up dwelling on it and the "infection" recurs over and over. When looking for which emotion is lodged where and the client wants to know when and what caused it, I suggest you give them only the age at which it occurred and who the interaction was with. Most of the time, they have a good idea what the incident was and won't dwell on it.

I know when I did a discovery on my allergies and was looking for a reason, it brought up such repulsive thoughts that it made my issue worse. Just a warning.

I use a table of emotions and where they might be lodged. (A good one is from "The Emotion Code" by Dr. Bradley Nelson.) I don't see any reason to reinvent the wheel. On that table, which you can view at http://scientifichealer.com/book-bonus/, you'll also see a list of organs where the emotions could be lodged. There is also a "heart-wall" that Dr. Nelson mentions in his book, he shows how to go about removing the wall, which is a barrier to your heart. Those of us who were in dysfunctional families with a lot of criticism and illogical actions tend to build them up. You may also be born with them.

Once your buried emotion and its location is discovered, send a grounding cord from the base of your spine to the center of the Earth, just as it says in the guided meditation. Make it nice and wide and let everything go. Let all the excess energy drain out of your body. If you can't feel the release, then test for it via muscle testing, until you are 100% clear of the excess energy. Now attach a line of energy from the body part, gland, organ, or system to the main grounding cord. Start "tapping" out the low energy emotion from the affected area with a motion of your hand, as if you're gently coaxing it out of your body. You may feel it leaving via a flow of energy in that area, a tingling, or just a feeling of relief. For everyone, the experience feels different. Sometimes, I get a tingling sensation, as if the area is being energized again after being asleep. Don't be alarmed if you feel nothing. Many don't but it is still occurring. Often, after the clearing is complete, those that felt nothing will remark their mood is better or some other upbeat comment.

The next step is to start sending in bright energy symbolically, a bright nearly white light with a gold tinge to it. Keep pumping that in until you test that the affected area is saturated. If you're sensitive, you'll feel a huge relief and even exhilaration.

Once you've cleared the first one, look for another two to three emotions to clear. Best practice is not to do more than 3 or 4 emotions at any one sitting because the shift will be too large and may send the client (or yourself) into a healing crisis where the symptoms are worse for a while until they get better. It's best to avoid that. You can muscle test when it is enough.

Exercise, listen to the guided meditation before going to sleep every night. Imagine while listening that you attach all your organs to your grounding cord and let the various low energy emotions go down the grounding cord. This promotes a restful sleep.

Practice and reading: Dr. Bradley Nelson, The Emotion Code. http://scientifichealer.com/emotion-code

Listen to the guided healing audio daily as it contains not only grounding and clearing for excess energy but also a grounding and clearing of emotions from the organs.

http://diamondhealingmethod.com

photo by Ferran Jorda, 2007

7. Your relationships play a key role in your health

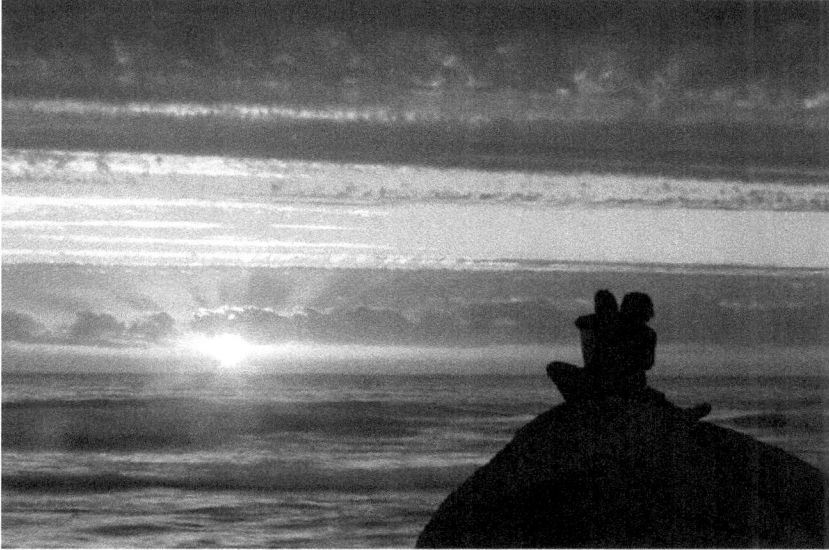

"Stress should be a powerful driving force, not an obstacle."
Bill Phillips

Core to our existence is our relationships

The quality of your life hinges on the quality of your relationships. The better you are able to connect with people, the more successful you'll be in life. If you are in a marriage or in business, your relationships will be everything. The same goes for your peace of mind, your financial success, and your success in love.

Our relationships reflect who we are at the moment. We likely have come into this life and chosen our particular family or constellation to learn and work through the issues that we want to overcome. There are a number of people who firmly believe this concept, that we choose our families and people we are to interact with. Many people describe to me that when they met certain people, there was a familiarity and they became fast friends/lovers almost immediately. While I'm not going to argue the truth of these statements, I am going to say that the Diamond Method protocol helps alleviate the stresses of relationships, how ever they came into being.

Now you understand that low energy emotions locked into your body can deplete you to the point of causing an illness or disease in that area. They can also sensitize you to situations that can cause difficulties in relationships. It can also be a vicious cycle: your relationships may cause you difficulties in your emotional life.

Once your emotions are clear, however, you might find that you still are trapped in repeating behavior that you no longer want with someone close to you in your life. It might be something you feel compelled to continue even though it makes no sense. This may be related to an agreement or contract you made with that person either before or during this lifetime. Or it may be a karmic relationship. In any case, you are energetically tied to someone in some way, shape or form.

Let me define relationships; these can be in any capacity. It can be a parent to child, a sibling, an aunt or uncle to niece or nephew, a significant other, a business relationship, an important friend, or anyone you have a karmic connection with, no matter how big or small.

Your difficult relationships are the ones you learn the most from. It is where you need to go if you are to progress and discover your true nature and who you are. If you were already confident, accepting of yourself, aware of your true nature, you wouldn't be in the difficult relationship. They are there to teach you those things.

Most people that end a difficult relationship and haven't resolved any issues will re-create the same situation again and again. They'll even wonder if all men (or women) are exactly the same because they keep ending up in a similar situation. Only the names and faces have changed. It's not the others; it is you that hasn't changed. You will keep attracting the thing you need to learn the most. If you don't learn it, you will keep attracting the lesson until you do. It's human nature to try to solve it.

The time to leave a relationship is when you feel there's closure with it. It's a calm acceptance that you have both done everything in your power to get through the struggle and resolve it. Sometimes it is meant to be only short term, sometimes it isn't. So many people feel guilty or confused that a relationship has ended. Some feel ashamed, especially if it is the first time in a family that someone has divorced or that there are children involved. Relationships can be difficult but fortunately not all of them are.

Some people fit together like hand in glove and get along because they are in a similar place on their path. They vibrate at the same frequency, or are on the same wavelength, so to speak. They get each other, even if their behavior doesn't seem the healthiest. They have agreed to work things through, love each other no matter what, and live out their lives together. They progress at a similar rate, sometimes one moves ahead and the other catches up. They are still making progress but usually at a slower rate.

Some of us are in a hurry and take the difficult road of difficult and painful relationships. Sometimes the lesson needs to be to discover who you really are and that no one can put you down, only you can put you down. It is you that is accepting the poor treatment. It stops when you decide it will. You then discover ways to expect only good behavior from others and then you find that's exactly what you get.

In all cases, your relationships are there to help you become who you are meant to be and those people that took up that role in your life need to be thanked. They took a role that didn't make them feel good either. You are each dancing around the other in ways that don't feel good at all. But the lesson can only come through opening you up, exposing the soft emotional side of you and learning that you are more than those painful feelings that you have.

Gratitude is the answer to finding closure

There are many situations in history that propelled someone to greatness due to great challenge. Those that provided the challenge were just as important as those that prevailed over them. How could someone be recognized for bringing peace to a world if there was no war? How could someone be a savior if there was no persecution? How can someone put forth a great scientific discovery if there was no one doubting it? We could name several instances in history where there was an antagonist egging someone on.

In the case of Isaac Newton, it was Robert Hooke. In the case of Jesus, it was Judas. The many harsh and often acerbic critiques of works of art, science, literature, politics, and music, etc., propelled the creator of the works to greater heights. We've seen this happen over and over again, no matter what the field of work. The critics are to be thanked for their job as each time they give an honest and constructive (or even difficult to take) assessment; it is up to the creators to decide if it has merit and either improve it or decide that their work can stand on its own.

It is the same with you and relationships. The difficult ones do propel you, they get you to think, and they get you to react in all sorts of ways. In all cases, you are constantly assessing: is my behavior okay or not, are my actions okay or not, is what I did constructive or destructive, is this relationship worth staying in or not, will I allow this sort of behavior towards me or not? There is a constant sorting, assessing, deciding, and thinking about what is happening, especially when things are difficult. None of us gives up easily on a relationship we've invested time in and so ending one is just as difficult as staying in it.

Is it over if it's over?

If, when ending a relationship, you are still angry at one another, the relationship is not over. You are still going to carry each other's energies around. Neither of you are ready for anything new until everything has run its course and you can look at one another in gratitude or at the worst neutrality. There can be no regret, anger, sorrow, disgust, jealousy, fear, anxiety, or other low energy emotion. If that is there, your energies are still entwined and affecting each of you. In the next section, you'll learn how to dissipate those energies. Without releasing them, your hands aren't empty, they're still full and you can't receive anything new or worthwhile while you are still in an emotional dance with your old relationship.

Because someone played the role for you that allowed you to learn, advance, and develop, your response, rather than a negative emotion, should be gratitude. It took me a while to get there after I divorced my children's father. I knew that without him, I wouldn't have my wonderful children or grandchild, I knew that my career would have run a less favorable course, and I knew that I wouldn't be who I am now without him.

But to come to that peaceful place and look at him with fondness and gratitude, it required me to clear out the old emotions and ties I had in that relationship. For nearly twenty years, I couldn't form a new significant relationship until I cleared out our energetic baggage with one another. When that happened, it was like magic, we, my ex- and I, reached a new level of friendship with one another, one of warmth and kindness. Subsequently, I found a new wonderful relationship and married.

Let's see how this letting go with gratitude, love and appreciation can proceed. In the next section, you'll discover the symbolic keys for uncoupling any relationship. It can even be a relationship you keep but want to stop certain compulsive actions or change the dynamics in the relationship.

How to clear relationships of old harmful baggage:

These procedures work whether you are working to cut the ties with someone but still have emotional baggage left over, are wanting to change your interaction with someone but still intend to keep them in your life, or have just met someone and want to make sure there's no baggage from a past life interaction. In all cases, it allows you to come to emotional peace within any relationship.

I learned from a healing teacher than I should clear all relationships as a matter of course. But in my own testing, I found this is not always necessary. It's only necessary if there's a negative emotional charge associated with it. Important people that I've cleared include my daughter, my mother, my ex's, and a few other difficult people in my life. It amounts to about a dozen. When I asked if I needed to clear my relationship with my husband, it came up a "no". We seem to be very much in tune with one another, we approach each other with generosity, kindness, and love. It is unlikely, but if that should change, I have a tool at my disposal that can correct the problem.

I understand that all people in my life tend to be a mirror to hold up to myself so I can see who I am. If I see something in someone else, that means I have that quality within myself. I wouldn't be able to see it otherwise. This is why dishonest people think everyone is cheating them and why honest people are easy marks for crooks to take advantage of.

Understanding this principle can really help you look at someone who is annoying you with new understanding. What trait does that annoying person have that is causing your annoyance? Is there something about you that is similar or that you might be worried about? These are questions I ask myself when I run across someone like that.

Yolanda was one such person. She teaches foreigners. She loves their stories and wants to highlight them to other people so they may be inspired. When she is in a room full of people, she'll command their attention, but in a very forward and annoying way. So many people don't want to deal with her. She irritates them to no end. And she may or may not be aware of this. I seem to not be annoyed by her but I can feel the reaction of others when she speaks, one of the drawbacks of being empathic.

My read on Yolanda is that she is protective of her inner core and doesn't let anyone in. She's insecure and wants approval from other people. She has a braggy style and this is what puts people off. No one who is secure within himself needs validation from others. Because I respect and applaud her actions in helping other people, I actually see her for who she really is, she relaxes and becomes more open with me and she allows a connection because she feels safe. She is one person who would greatly benefit from getting some of her emotional baggage cleared out, particularly from old hurtful relationships. She would then be able to connect with others with confidence because she would feel safe and secure around anyone.

The first step, reclaiming your energy

Whenever you interact with anyone, there is an exchange of "energy." "Energy" can take the form of information, emotion, thoughts, healing, curses, or physical form such as massage. In conversation, when one person yields the lion's share of the information and the other collects it, there is an energy imbalance and the person doing all the talking and sharing will end up tired at the end of the conversation. If you are a teacher, you will feel much the same way if there is not a fair exchange and dialog during your class time. It doesn't matter what the interaction is, whether it is with the cashier at the store, your coworker or your child, there is energy exchanged.

The trouble with the exchange and sharing of other people's energy is that it mixes in with our own. Nearly everyone's personal energy is at a slightly different frequency than ours and it vibrates in our bodies. As you continue to accumulate all those foreign energies, it causes a long-term degradation of our own because the waves destructively interfere with one another. The solution is to clear out those energies. You can reclaim your energy back from others and give them back theirs using a symbolic ritual. Some people would call it a soul retrieval. It basically means that you don't have to keep tabs on everyone else, you only need to tend to yourself. It's like weeding your own garden as opposed to tending everyone else's and letting yours get messy in the process.

In long term and deep relationships, the exchange of energy is much more profound. In this case, a separate small ritual is performed in which the other's energy is drawn out from you and vice versa. Your energy from the other is then cleaned up and brought back to you and that of the other is given back to him/her. The energies are cleaned up and exchanged by storing the in a symbol. Remember, the mind and thoughts are very powerful: using the symbols helps the subconscious understand and participate to bring about the desired results.

For the cleansing, I use the symbol of the rose with my clients, which to me symbolizes love and purity. The rose draws out your energy from the other, cleans it up and allows it to flow back into you. The results from this process have been profound for some clients. They experience a renewed energy for their life and are able to experience life with a renewed vigor.

Angela, a 50-year-old woman living near the beach, was one such person. The last decade had her feeling weaker and more tired than ever before. She came to me because she had brain surgery to remove a tumor, which had made her feel terrible before the surgery. She was listless, could barely get herself out of the house not even to visit the ocean which was always her favorite place to be, and she felt terrible being a burden to her husband, whom she dearly loved.

She was a generous person and contributed to everyone's lives without leaving much for herself. After giving her a tune-up and clearing out most other issues, it still remained that she had too much of other people's energy in her body. Using the rose to absorb foreign energies, I helped retrieve her energy from all the people in her life that she had given it away to and removed everyone else's energy from her body. The transformation was nothing short of miraculous. She now has the energy to go out and exercise daily at the shore to her great joy, be a great partner to her husband, and is enthusiastic about her life again.

In a relationship clearing, the first step is to retrieve your energy from the other and give them back theirs.

Energetic cords allow exchange of energy

Any significant relationship creates energetic connections or cords between you. The cords can connect at various parts of the body. They typically connect at the heart, the solar plexus and the sacral area. Some connect at the third eye and some at the root area.

When they connect at the root and a relationship ends badly, you will have an energetic drain on your ability to provide for yourself. You may even have money bleeding out in places and you can't quite figure out why this is happening. If you are connected at the sacral area, it is usually with a significant other. You may feel zero sex drive, lose your creativity, and not want to partner with anyone new. At the solar plexus, you may lose your confidence, you may feel drained of energy, and/or you may have a lot of anger or disappointment. At the heart area, you'll hurt or feel sad about your relationship. That will also drain you of energy. At the head, you could become foggy headed and not be able to think clearly or lose your intuitive sense.

The first procedure is cutting those cords; only the negative cords will be cut with a relationship you intend keeping, such as a parent or child. Ask express permission when doing so. When this happens, the cords leave a hole in your energy field and will drop automatically away from the other person. The holes in your field need to be resealed or the cords will reform even when not wanted. If you intend to keep the relationship, you can also form new cords but only after you've cleared your contracts and agreements and complete the karmic connection between you.

This is the process I use, which is something I've heard over again over the years of learning healing. My most recent healing teacher reminded me of it again. By cutting these energetic cords, you stop the bleeding of energy from you to another and vice versa. This way you can learn to draw on the infinite supply of external energy on your own and stop depending on everyone else for it. Likewise, you can block the person drawing from you.

The easiest way to do this process without learning the process in detail is to use the guided meditation for clearing relationships. It guides you through the process. (http://scientifichealer.com/audios) As you listen, imagine them dropping off you and the cord disappearing from sight. The cord automatically drops away once it no longer carries energy. Now seal up all those places on your body (or that of your client) using a "spiritual cement of sorts". This will help keep the cords from forming again until you invite them in. You just imagine the places sealing up and forming a hard edge to protect yourself.

Smooth out your aura/energy field. Now you are ready to have your contracts and agreements dissolved.

Dissolving contracts and agreements

Contracts and agreements are slightly different in the context of relationships. A contract is a marriage where you agree to be each other's legal partners. An agreement might be the way you agree to treat each other, such as, "I am your husband; you shall obey me." It could also be, "I am your husband, I will protect you and provide for you."

In the context of a business relationship, for example, a contract would be the various roles you take on in the partnership, as legally prescribed. An agreement would be how you carry out the partnership.

It doesn't matter how simple the agreement. Let's say someone tells you, "let's get together and do lunch sometime." You agree. This constitutes an agreement. Not upholding it makes gives that agreement energy and it binds you to that person until you fulfill or dissolve the agreement.

As you learned in Chapter 5, words matter. You need to mind your words and if you blurt out something you don't mean, say something, such as "cancel, cancel" to allow yourself to take it back. Agreeing to something you don't intend to fulfill is just as inauthentic as telling a lie.

You can dissolve the binding of contracts and agreements by imagining that you have a key in your pocket. Imagine drawing it out and you look down and see that your arm or leg is shackled to that contract/agreement. Unlock the shackle with the key and let the chain fall off. Let all of it drop down a grounding cord that goes down to the center of the Earth.

In the next step, imagine the agreements or contracts as documents whose print spells out the details of the relationship and are signed by both parties.

In dissolving them, you first determine how many of each type you have between the two of you, say one contract and two agreements. Then you have the printed /signed documents before you in your mind's eye hovering between you, in this case it would be three. As you pump universal energy into the contracts and agreements, you dissolve the agreements as you watch the print and signatures fade off the paper. Once all the papers are blank sheets of paper, the contracts and agreements are dissolved.

Completing the Karmic Cycle

Often it is said that we come into life with agreements with our spiritual family members to learn certain lessons and to experiment with different constellations. We might come across people that we "know" even thought we've never met them physically before. They feel familiar, we click with them instantly and we become fast friends, lovers, partners, and spouses. I've met several couples that admitted to me that they agreed to marry within days of meeting each other for the first time. They stayed married for decades and happily so. We can also wander around life decades and not have this experience.

Sometimes the constellation that we agreed upon becomes too much to handle and we dissolve the relationship before we've completed this karmic agreement. Sometimes the agreement causes us difficulty in a relationship we want to keep and move past the previous one. In this case, completing the karmic cycle has brought a great deal of relief to people wanting to be done with the old connection and just move on.

Again, this work is symbolic, much like the agreements/contracts. In the case of dissolving the karma, we want to change and recycle that energy. As the guided meditation tells you, you imagine the person you wish to clear Karma with seated across from you, 30 to 50 feet away. This is close enough for you to know who it is but far enough away that you can't hear anything being said. Halfway between the two of you grows a rose up out of the ground. It is huge, two feet in diameter. Its petals are bright white. The rose is the symbol of love and purity; it can absorb and purify the karmic energy. As the rose has fully bloomed, you see a ring aligned vertically start to form directly above it. The ring represents the karma between the two of you. The top half of the ring starts to solidify into a gold half ring. This represents the karma you have already experienced with this person.

The ring will begin to fill in, and it continues during this process. When it is complete, the karmic circle you had with that person is now complete. As the ring is completed, solid and gold, it drops into the middle of the white rose, which closes around the ring, engulfing it and absorbing the karmic energy. As this occurs, turn the rose and ring into dust and let it drop down the root hole all the way to the center of the Earth. The Earth will take the energy and purify and recycle it. It no longer exists in its former form.

Now that you've completed what you set out to do with that person, he or she stands up, waves goodbye or blows you a kiss, turns around and walks off into the distance and fades out away from you. Thank them for being in your life and doing what needed to be done to help you become the person you were always meant to be. If you can't let go in love and gratitude, let go in neutrality. This completes the clearing of your relationship.

Now you may choose to reform a relationship but the connections will be unlike the old. Your relationship with your child who is now an adult can go from parent-child to adult-adult, for example. Or go from ex-spouses at odds to two good friends that know they don't make it as a couple.

There is one other aspect of relationships that needs to be addressed, that of protecting yourself from the negative or destructive energies of people that will work to draw yours down.

Protecting yourself from negative energies

Before I start on the draining nature of negative energies, I'd like to ask you this question. Have you ever walked into a room and felt an amazing warmth and energy and knew that it came from someone that seemed to light up the room? This person is aware of their Divine nature and brings in the infinite universal energy and it flows outward towards everyone. This is someone who is generous with their spirit, and is balanced and happy.

Often, people aren't aware of their divine nature nor are they aware of the infinite amount of energy available to them. Instead, they will draw from the personal energy of the people around them. They are tiresome in their neediness to most of the people around them. Some people are drawn in by their neediness because they feel useful and that person supplies them with those good feelings. Some people call the needy people energy vampires. In the long haul, the person catering to the needy person is the one that gets ill and dies early because you can't serve the needs of two people all the time: yourself and that other person.

Sometimes, whole families operate on these principles and it is very difficult to live within the family culture. "Going home" again feels like an endless drain of your personal energy and resources. In this case, just clearing the energy flow between you and the other person isn't enough. If you are in proximity and sometimes even if you're not, you will feel drained around those people. Often, their words can also affect you as you have already learned. Often this is more important than the energy issues with a needy person.

Here are two ways to set up a barrier between you and the person or people that are affecting you. You can try each way to see which one is suited for you.

The first method is to pull your energy field in close to you, eighteen inches is a good distance instead of the usual 3 feet. This is mentioned in the healing audio at http:// diamondhealingmethod.com. This keeps their energy field out of yours as much as possible. The next thing to do is to put a hard edge on the outside edge of your energy field. Make it like Plexiglas or hard crystal. You can tint it a blue or blue green color that is a protective filter color. This type of filter is known as a band pass filter in the laboratory; it's effective at cutting out the low energy emotions and thoughts such as anger, jealously, hate, sorrow, and fear. It allows in the high-energy thoughts and emotions of joy, love, happiness, and peace.

The next method is to create a quantum bubble around you. The way you find out how this feels is to find a quantum scalar device and get near it. If you don't feel its calmness, your body does. You can mimic this by drawing universal energy around your body and intend the energy barrier to mimic the field. You'll see such a device pictured below.

You don't need to buy one, just mimic one. If you ever meet me, ask me for mine and I'll show you and demo the making of the field. Use the same blue green color to coat the edge of the field. This has been so effective that the number of headaches, number of issues involving others, and other invasion problems has decreased dramatically amongst my clients.

You can also use two simple symbolic techniques. One is to bring down a chopping motion in front of your body as if your cutting connecting cords. Do this three times if someone is trying to engage you in a negative discourse. Another is to bring a symbolic zipper from pubic bone to the top of your head. Imagine it a few inches in front of your body. Do this three times and it will stop negative thoughts from others and you won't absorb them and become weak.

Tribal Beliefs

Other ways your family of origin relationships affect you are what you were told when you were very young and you internalized it. When you are young, you are not capable of processing certain pieces of information; you just store it. You are told that boys don't cry or girls must be gracious and polite at all times, girls can't do math, boys must be in a sport, or that everyone in the family plays music. These are the typical ones.

You'll also hear your parents reflect their belief system: money didn't make them any happier, you have to work hard for your money, the road to hell is paved with good intentions, money doesn't grow on trees, and money is the root of all evil. You have religious mores and beliefs, such as needing to fast on Fridays, needing to go to church once a week, needing to go to confession, or saying so many hail Mary's if you've done something that you weren't supposed to. We all grow up with these kinds of things and it's often difficult to outgrow them even if they don't fill our needs any more.

It's basic programming to your subconscious. It doesn't help that none of the statements above are true; these are just other people's rules. They do not have to do with honoring yourself, your family, your higher power/God, or your planet. They are just rules that are constructed to help you put structure around your life, as most children need structure to feel safe and secure. In reality, because many of those rules are not "truth", they will make your muscles go weak as you read in Chapter 3. They are not life sustaining, they cause your body undue stress. Think about this. Every day of your life that you maintain and live by rules that are not life sustaining exerts constant stress, which over the long haul accumulates physical and emotional damage in the body.

For example, there's a boy who wants to express his feelings and cry. As an adult, he remains stoic even at a good friend's funeral and poopoos everyone else who is crying in grief for having lost him/her. Let's see what happens by looking at a real life situation.

In this true life example, Bud, a former captain in the Marines and a member of my family, remained stoic at his best friend's funeral. His friend Frank had died of lymphoma at the young age of 30. Frank's wife, Linda, was giving the most moving speech about the bravery that Frank showed while going through hellish chemotherapy treatments. How he loved her and their friends so much; she was reading the messages he left for them all. His last words to them were: his life was so wonderful because of the wonderful people in it. Go out from here and remember that.

There was not a dry eye in the house, except Bud's. He leaned over to me and whispered as I wept openly. He said, "You aren't going to cry, too, are you?" I looked at him squarely in the eye and said, "yes, I sure am!"

This was typical for Bud. He never showed his emotions or feelings, you didn't know what he was thinking, he was the perfect stoic Marine, and exactly as his parents brought him up to be, a boy that doesn't cry.

Fast forward 25 years, Bud never married, as he couldn't get close to any woman. He was handsome and most definitely heterosexual. But unable to express his feelings, he remained alone. Holding in his grief kept that energy locked down in his body. Grief, as mentioned in Chapter 5, the low energies resonating in the heart area affecting lungs, heart and thymus, deplete them of the life giving energy they need to repair and thrive.

Bud, then 56, was out hiking with a good friend. It was nothing strenuous, just a walk. Holding in the sadness and grief took its toll on his heart. During the walk, he sat down as he became weary and his heart gave out and he died within minutes with no way to save him. The problem with suppressing emotions is that you suppress all of them, not just the grief. It is a true story and I still grieve for his loss, as he was too young to die. Meanwhile, the irony of it is his parents, now in their nineties, are still alive.

Reprogramming tribal and religious beliefs

How do we reprogram ourselves to undo the religious and tribal programming? One of the problems with this kind of programming is that it is hard to undo once it is programmed in. Many people are afraid to question it, to get into conflict with the status quo. They're afraid because they think they'll be rejected. They've held those beliefs for so long that they think that they'll look foolish changing their minds.

You don't need to have any of those fears at all. Those that discard the mantle of popular belief and go with real truth start to stand in their own power. They become internally driven. There is something magnetizing about those people; you are naturally attracted to them. In addition, if you are internally driven, you will model it for other people and they will match you. You will help shift them towards also becoming internally driven. The real truth is that you are a powerful creator, that the relatively arbitrary and even punitive rules that most of us have lived by don't serve you any more.

To overcome the old programming, talk therapy has usually been the answer. How else do we reprogram what we've been told except to talk to someone about how all those rules don't work for you any more. Not surprising is that even after years of talk therapy, the client is not much further along than they were when they started. They go, dredge up the past, even cry about it, and don't take any steps to move forward. They get upset again, go in and talk about it, get relieved, and go out and continue life as before. The undoing or reprogramming requires an energetic shift. It is more successful if the client is able to take action.

There are a couple of common issues that I've come across that hold people back. One is that they forget that **love is a gift**. You don't have to earn it. Look at how a child feels about the parent. You can be the worst parent in the world, but your child will still love you. You did not earn that love, you receive it because you are. Another misconception is that your abundance is separate from your love. Your love is your abundance. Your health, wealth and relationships are all proportional to the love you have for yourself and others.

To remove tribal and common beliefs takes practice until you've arrived at mastery. Here are suggested steps to do this on your own:

1. Listen to a guided meditation or meditate daily.
2. Start a practice of gentle yoga, one that stimulates the twelve meridians of the body. Gentle stretches and poses that you hold will activate your body in positive ways. Doing it quietly will allow you to reflect, get reacquainted with your physical self, and make you more mindful of your being.
3. Write or find a set of daily affirmations that speak to programming yourself to accept and love you just as you are. You have to remember that you are on a spiritual path to learn about your true nature. You are discarding all the things that aren't you to find your true essence and nature. Here are some suggestions you might begin with:

- I love and accept myself unconditionally.
- I am perfect as I am, that I am in exactly the right place to be exactly who I am meant to be.
- I acknowledge my accomplishments and the effort and courage it took to achieve them.
- I recognize the divinity in me. I respect myself and treat myself with kindness and love.
- I accept myself for what I am. My path is to continue on this journey of self-discovery.
- I am a valuable person and I am pleasing and helpful to the people around me.
- I am worthy.
- I am my own best friend.
- I treat myself as if I am the most valuable person in the

world.
- I am loved for who I am.

4. Fix yourself healthy meals daily.

5. Make a gratitude list every morning and say it out loud.

If you still feel stuck, it's time to bring in the outside help of someone that can guide you through the process. If not me, then one of my apprentice healers who have been trained to do this. Please call at 310-692-4036 or contact me at http://scientifichealer.com/contact/

Photo by Thokrates, 2007

8. Your marvelous DNA, its incredible engineering

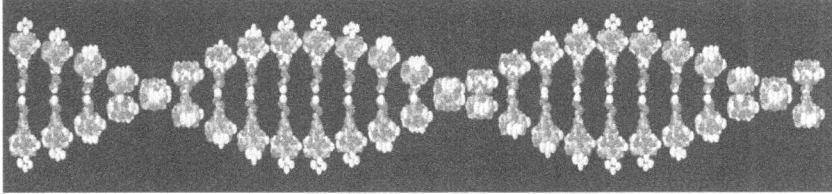

"Give yourself a break. When you are alone with your thoughts, you shouldn't be arguing."
Gary Rudz

You'll find in this chapter that we are often preprogrammed with how we manage stress by virtue of our birth into a family. We inherit habits and behavior without realizing it. It isn't in our energetic blueprint, instead it is stored in our DNA. Let's find out more about DNA and how we can reprogram it for our benefits.

Your body is an incredible piece of engineering.

You were born with the most incredible feat of engineering imaginable. Think about it. Our bodies have about 38 trillion cells in them. Yes, that's 38 with 12 zeros after it. To give you some idea of how much that is, if you take 38 trillion grains of sand (make them average size), you would end up with something over 40,000 tons. That's 80,000,000 pounds.

To imagine that visually, the USS Enterprise aircraft carrier only weighs 20,000,000 pounds. So, in other words, 38 trillion grains of sand weighs the same as 4 aircraft carriers. In comparison, an average sized male is only about 180 pounds. This comparison is mind-boggling.

The really fantastic and practically unbelievable part comes here. Each cell in your body undergoes about 9 trillion chemical reactions per day to sustain, energize, and repair itself. Multiply those by the 38 trillion cells, that's a whole lot of reactions in the body. Your body is doing all this without you even being aware of it. We are all walking miracles.

These reactions rejuvenate, heal, energize, restore, purify and keep us running even if we abuse our bodies. Our bodies are highly adaptable and complex, with redundant systems in place to keep us, that is our spirits, well-housed and functioning for a lot longer than it would seem possible.

Every cell in your body is a hologram

It is even more amazing to consider that in each cell, yes, all 38 trillion of them, there are 23 pairs of chromosomes with a total of 25,000 molecules containing 3 billion base pairs.

These coded words don't just contain the instructions for our eye color, hair color, height and other physical characteristics, they also tell us what our likes and dislikes are, our personality, our belief systems, what we inherited in terms of our character, penchants and basically where we fall in the scale of human vibration/emotional make-up.

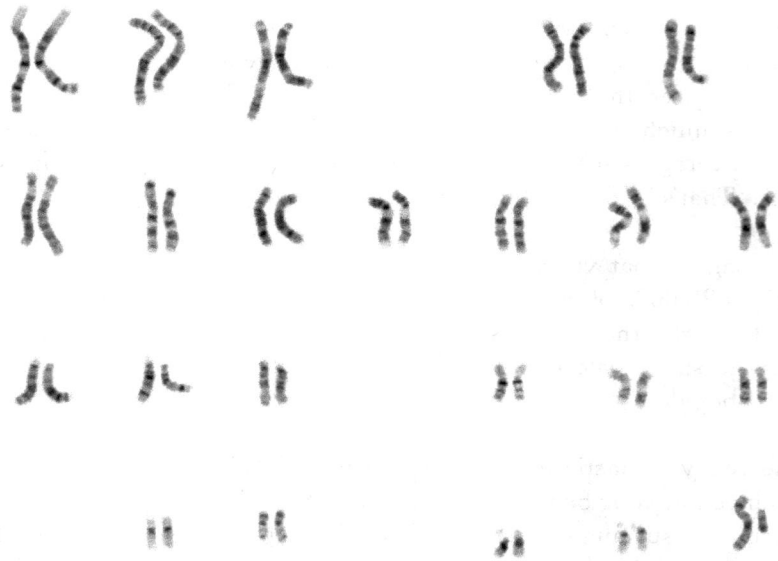

Above you see a representative photo of human chromosomes. This means that every single cell in our bodies has all the information it needs to make you from head to toe, like each piece of a hologram gives you the picture of the whole. Each cell also contains all the coding to make and keep you perfectly healthy, regenerate so you can last many years longer than you ever dreamed.

Our heritage, our DNA, is an incredible engineering marvel.

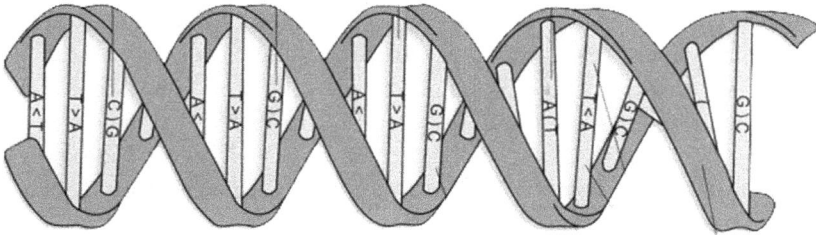

Your entire genetic code is in every cell of your body. A new physical body that is identical to your current body could ostensibly be created with the DNA information from any one cell from any part of your body. It is the reason that sometimes people claim that we are holograms because like a hologram, every part contains the information of the whole. What I just said might be confusing to some because we have so many different kinds of cells, so how is it that a red blood cell, a muscle cell and a liver cell have all the same coding information in their nuclei.

At conception we start with one cell, a combination of both parent's DNA. This is the master cell. As it divides, stem cells are created. In the beginning, all stem cells in your body are identical. A stem cell is one that instructs other cells how to grow and divide. If a stem cell is placed in a certain environment, such as a changing pH or temperature, it will differentiate according to the instructions encoded in the DNA. It all happens at the cell wall.

The cell wall transmits instructions to the DNA as to how the cell is to differentiate and what kind of tissue it's to become. Thus, the different types of cells were given specific instructions based on what environment they found themselves in to change from the original master cell, or zygote (a fertilized egg) to the specific kind of cell they end up as. The cell wall interprets the environment and transmits the information to the cell nucleus, which tells the DNA exactly how to produce which type of cell to produce.

Furthermore, it is said that our DNA predetermines about half our behavior as well as our physical appearance. It not only contains all the programming needed to produce all the protein in our bodies, it determines our eye color, hair color, height and skin color but also your propensity for certain diseases, your likes and dislikes, your attitudes towards abundance and wealth, and your ability to maintain a healthy relationship, to name a few.

This information is contained in the 15 to 20 thousand molecules in the human genome, which contains 3 billion pairs of nucleic bases along the chains that make them up. The chains are twisted into a double helix as shown in the image at left. The letters along the crossbars indicate the individual nucleic bases (guanine, adenine, thymine, and cytosine). Since each genetic "word" in the DNA chain consists of 3 pairs, that means that there are a billion pieces of information in the human genome. Unlike other species of fauna and flora, over 95 percent of our human DNA does not sequence proteins. Although there have been discoveries of what some of the rest of the pieces are doing, there is still a lot that isn't known.

Do you have "junk" DNA?

One of the main functions of DNA is to structure protein chains for use in your body. The separate amino acids attach to their specific 3 code sequence and line up along the DNA chain. Not all DNA sequences proteins. Since it isn't exactly clear what the balance of the structure does, many scientists call the non protein sequencing portion "junk DNA". What they are not comprehending is that there is nothing superfluous in the body and that DNA contains not just the information on how tall we are or the color of our eyes, but also carries the tribal and inherited traits such as basic spiritual beliefs, affinities, and things that might repulse you. It also contains tendencies like if you come from a family that is deeply religious or spiritual, you will likely have the same affinity.

For example, if you come from a family that has criminals, it might be hard to resist illegal activity or if you come from a family that has a lot of poverty, it would be hard to overcome that and become wealthy easily. One very common trait amongst the middle class is that you have to work hard for your money, a more or less protestant work ethic. These are typical of the information that is stored in your personal DNA. This kind of programming is called epigenetics, which is now an emerging science. The DNA is the hardware, while the programming is the software.

How much of your DNA needs changing?

Remember that there are about a billion pieces of information in the human genome. In most cases, the pieces of information that are causing an affinity towards one thing or another is less than one thousand. That means that 99.9999% of your DNA does not contain such information. At left, you can see the set of human chromosomes. If you total up all the non-desirable characteristics, it usually doesn't amount to more than 0.001% of your DNA coding. Looking at the positive: it means that 99.999% of your DNA is awesome and that we are only having to shift a very small proportion of it for your desired result.

You have to remember that the DNA you'd like to shift is neither "good" nor "bad". Let's look at a particular case. If your family tends to be overweight and have a very difficult time slimming down, it is very likely you are also struggling with this same issue. Years ago, when the food supply was less certain, this was a desirable characteristic because it meant that during famines, your family would survive and those that had to eat constantly to maintain their mass would not. The ones we envy now are the people that usually died off during the famines.

Now with a certain food supply, this characteristic is actually detrimental to our health as adding more fat to our bodies generally decreases our health in the form of high blood pressure, high cholesterol, more strain on the heart, less fitness and so forth. Obese people tend to die younger. What was a survival advantage is now a disadvantage.

Can DNA influences that are no longer serving you be removed?

There is a way to alter DNA physically. Scientists are now exploring this via genetic engineering for treatment of cancer. This is not the stem cell therapy I'll talk about shortly, but actually altering a gene sequence along the DNA strand. It is actually frightening to think they are altering only one area of the genome to cause a certain change in cell growth without exploring all the other areas that might be affected but they are successfully healing certain cancers using this technique. Fortunately, a Diamond Healing can remove the no longer desired influences on our being without going to such lengths, is safer in the hands of an experienced healer, and covers all portions of the stored information, not just in one location on the genome.

The basics are given here but for those that are not skilled at moving their own energy, either a guided meditation (available at http://scientifichealer.com/audios/), taking a class (such as the one offered at http://scientifichealer.com/course/), or a healer skilled in these methods could help you complete this process.

To start: Ground yourself and connect with the universal or divine energy above. Now you can imagine you are looking at your DNA all spread out. Remember it's 23 pairs of chromosomes and the images in this chapter give you a good idea of how they look. Imagine you are looking at these 23 pairs all lined up, let them unravel from the nucleus of your master cell in your mind's eye. The master cell started was when you were just a twinkle in your parents eye, the fertilized egg. If you are adept at muscle testing, you can test for how many pieces of DNA coding carries the information you want to change, let's say, a poverty mindset. You can also just look at the laid out genome and count up the pieces. Typically, it will be 100 to 500, but it can be more or less. Counting the pieces of information helps you gauge how deeply seated or intense the issue is and how much time you need to spend removing the influence.

While looking at your DNA in your mind's eye, ask that those pieces be made known to you and while you imagine where this information is sitting, letting it "light up" in some color. I use gray since the rest of the DNA will generally be a more vibrant color. Then "pluck" the information carrying the trait you want to clear off and replace it with "healthy" information. You can move your hand in a plucking motion: this is done energetically using a healing light: it can be cobalt blue or golden. Do not choose what information to replace it with but let it be divinely chosen simply because we are all too limited to imagine how expansive and incredible something new can be.

After the pieces with that trait are removed, roll the DNA back up into the nucleus of the master or stem cell and "seal" the healing into it by watching healing light shoot into it. Tell the body that the new programming is now in place, the old programming is obsolete (you can again use healing light to do this). The new programming will run from now on, so every morning when you wake up, the new programming is in place.

Is that all there is to removing DNA influences?

Briefly, the answer is no. You can guess that since we are complex beings, an open system so to speak, there are a large number of factors that influence our behavior as mentioned in an earlier chapter, including another DNA factor: that of belonging to your biological/spiritual family. We are all connected to this family DNA in some way energetically; this energetic connection can make it difficult to change your behavior even once your personal DNA in your body has been cleared of a particular factor or behavior.

The disconnection is simple but not always easy. For yourself, you have to decide whether you want to disconnect. If you are working on someone else, you have to make sure you have their express permission. Some people want to work through their own issues and do not want this part of them altered. Some of you may be wondering how this can be, but I have met people that when I asked whether I could clear this, their response was "no, I'm okay."

To disconnect you from your family DNA, ground yourself and connect with the Divine or universal energy. Now focus on the issue you want to clear and imagine that you are looking at your connection for this issue to a sphere containing your family DNA. You sever the energy flow using a chopping motion. Test as you're clearing until your connection shows to have a zero percent flow. You do not want to alter the family DNA bubble itself as each family member has to decide whether they want to be free of this issue or not. It is not our place to decide for other adults.

What factors of health or even my life can removing DNA influences affect?

You might be surprised to find out just how many factors of your life are found inside your DNA. I've alluded to some in the previous paragraphs. Here is a list but not an exhaustive one:
* remove inherited undesirable physical issues such as propensity towards a disease such as cancer, diabetes, obesity, Alzheimer's/dementia or high cholesterol. Some of these need to be corrected early enough to avoid long term damage that is hard to come back from.
* remove undesirable traits in behavior such as criminal activity, depression, anger impulses, self sabotaging behavior, self loathing, and/or poverty thinking.
* improve ability to have healthy, vibrant relationships instead of dysfunctional embattled ones.
* improve wealth and abundance by clearing DNA blocks to it - hard work ethic, not worthy, money is the root of evil, money doesn't grow on trees, etc.

What do stem cells have to do with it?

The news lately is full of research and new therapies with stem cells. A stem cell is a cell with all your encoding information that can differentiate to any cell in your body. Briefly, your stem cells are stored all over your body and are called progenitor cells. Stem cell therapy has been common for leukemia and other bone marrow problems where stem cells are extracted from healthy bone marrow and then the patient is treated with chemotherapy, which kills everything. The stem cells are introduced into the body to promote healthy cell growth.

Stem cell or gene therapy is now being experimented on for brain trauma, cancer, spinal cord injuries, baldness, deafness, ALS (Lou Gehrig's disease), diabetes, blindness, and even missing teeth. Stem cells are the crux of a Diamond Healing session and can even be released into the bloodstream to find the ailing cells to repair and rejuvenate that part of the body.

During the stem cell process, the recipients usually feel an energy surge so great that some of them feel like they need to sit or lie down, it's so overpowering. By releasing them, it allows the raw stem cells to attach to an ailing body part, particularly a cancerous one, and give it the correct instructions for replication. Several clients have reported rapidly shrinking tumors after this procedure.

None of the work is done to "fight" cancer. Instead, the body is boosted and the cells grow like they're supposed to. Cancerous tumors still contain your cells, they just forgot how to grow properly mainly because they've been exposed to some toxin and the body is unable to handle it. The stem cell protocol gives them the correct instructions. It may be only symbolic but it seems to be effective. I have not worked with anyone that it did not work on.

Juliet came to me after being given a dire diagnosis of inoperable lung cancer. She had "beaten" it once years before but it came back with a vengeance the second time. The tumor grew rapidly and the doctors had given her weeks to live. After a first set of profound healings, Juliet thrived for approximately a year.

At the one-year mark, I called her and said that I had the intuition to get in touch with her. She was weak, tired and emotionally drained, not just because her nodules started to grow again, but because she was in a toxic situation with her daughter. Her daughter had taken her in and it wasn't going well with both daughter and son-in-law. Juliet was a true believer in superb nutrition, meditation, and self-care, but for some reason, the energies flowing between her and her daughter were draining and she was exhausted. Her body was giving up because strife with her daughter was so painful to her.

When I spoke with Juliet, her voice was weak and quiet, and she felt defeated. I considered Juliet to be a beautiful light in the world and told her so. After being in a toxic situation, a loving voice is always good for anyone. Just as a matter of practice, find something kind to say to those around you. You'll watch the energy shift, stress calm down, and moods elevate each time. It does you as much good as those you compliment or even acknowledge.

The toxic situation brought Juliet's adrenal glands to near failure; her hypothalamus and pituitary were not functioning well. The cancer nodules in her lungs were growing. After helping her replenish those parts of her body that were failing (it included clearing her relationship with her daughter and son-in-law, grounding out feelings of guilt and sorrow, and changing her belief system about mothers and daughters), her bone marrow was stimulated to release stem cells throughout her body. They don't need direction, they are holographic as you've read about already. They give directions to whichever cells they find based on their environment.

Generally, during this process, the person on the receiving end gets a jolt of energy or a "buzz" from the release of energy in their body. Juliet was no different. On that day, she stood up from her bed renewed and ready to go. She felt so much better that she took the class that I offer to teach basic energy management techniques and started doing them herself.

DNA healing can also make your cells younger from the inside out

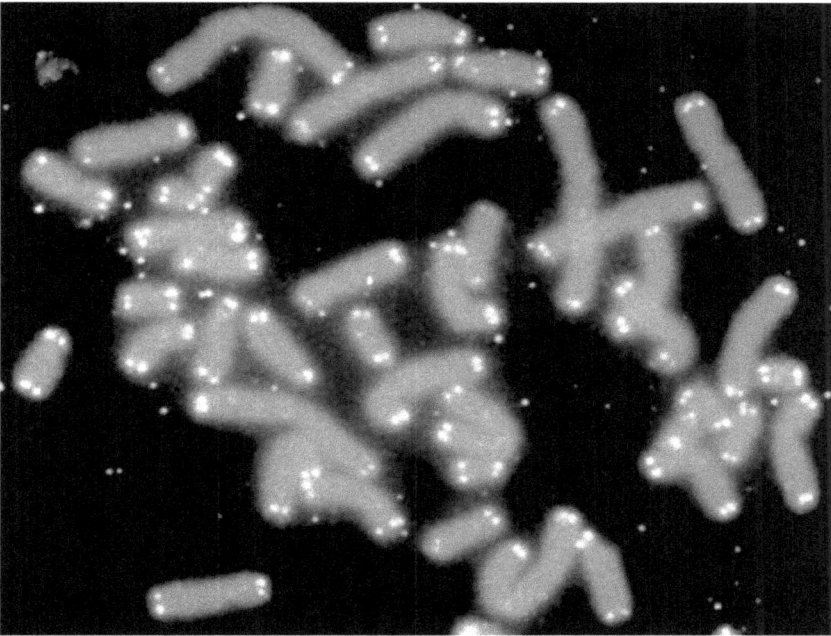

There is a rejuvenation process that involves the ends of the DNA strands. On the end of each chromosome is a single strand series of DNA that protects the integrity of the information sequencing along the double helix that have caught a lot of attention from the press relating to premature aging: the telomeres. Above, you'll find an image of human chromosomes with their telomeres lit up. This single strand shortens with each replication and even more so if you abuse your body with drugs, stress, alcohol and poor food choices. New research has shown that moving to nurturing and affirming health choices can actually lengthen the telomeres in your cells.

Below, you'll also find a cartoon of one of your chromosomes, which shows exactly how this single stranded extension of your DNA appears. This single strand curls up and forms the end-cap on the chromosome. When this telomere is gone, the DNA information becomes compromised. The cell replication starts from the centers of the strands, so the protein replication can work for a while but only partially. Eventually, the protein functionality (which includes enzymes, muscles, skin, organs, glands, bone marrow, hair, nails, etc.) will decrease and cease to be replicated properly. Before then, the function of the affected areas decreases due to lack of energy and lack of the proper amino acid sequences.

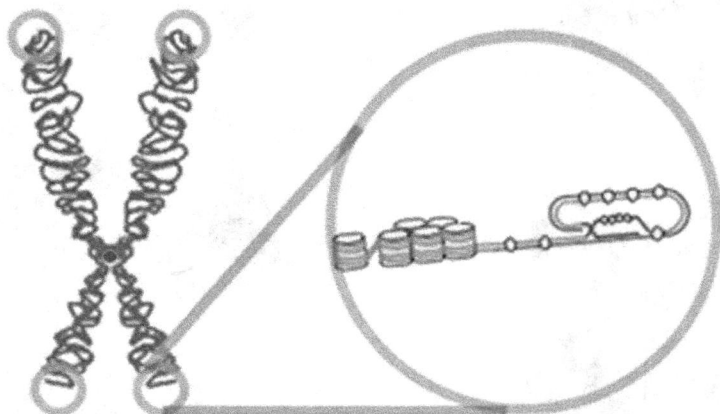

In the cellular rejuvenation process, the telomere is restored energetically. To do this, again you and/or the person being healed is grounded and connected to the Divine first. Then activate the stem or master cell for that part of your body, whether it is a system, gland or organ. You do this by first clearing and re-energizing the cell walls, the nucleus, and the organelles that help support the absorption of nutrients for the cell and the ejection of waste material, and the synthesis of protein. Then the telomeres are re-lengthened. Finally the cell is energized with healing energy throughout. At this point, the master or stem cell is ready to instruct the other cells in the affected area how to reproduce to younger versions of themselves.

You reflect this information across the entire system, gland or organ until as many of the cells respond as possible. You can test how much and how long the new cell growth will occur, but it is not necessary except to ask if more than 75% of the cells responded. If not, another such rejuvenation should be done in the not too distant future.

At this point, the cell rejuvenation is complete. This type of rejuvenation is most sensitive to abuse of the body, meaning too much alcohol, recreational drugs, junk food, lack of sleep, stress, and lack of exercise. Keeping thoughts optimistic, avoiding bloody, violent programs, and reducing stress through a number of techniques will go a long way to optimize the healing. See the post healing health-affirming steps after a healing and basically for your life in Chapter 10.

Conclusion

Your fate doesn't have to be the same as your parents or anyone else in your family. It is yours to choose as you desire. Altering the few DNA programs in your cells that are sabotaging your goals and desires, is a simple process but needs to be exercised with caution. If you've been healed in other areas, the DNA programs need to align with those healings or it could revert back to the same old patterns or condition. Conventional medical intervention is often like taking a sledge hammer to a problem that only needs a slight tap with your finger. The irony is that often, natural healing is the last resort after conventional medical care: it should be the first.

Photo by Mehmet Pinarci, 2014

9. The connection: allergies - autoimmune disorder

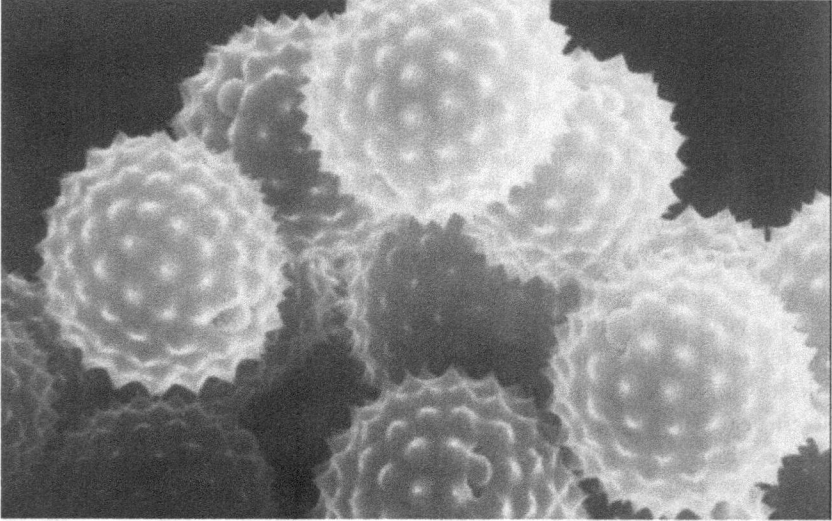

"For fast acting relief, try slowing down."
Lily Tomlin

Do you have a health problem that no one seems to be able to solve?

Maybe it's commonplace like high blood pressure or high cholesterol? What about arthritis, fibromyalgia, fatigue, depression or anxiety? How about hypothyroidism or adrenal failure? Maybe you weigh way too much. Did you know all these things can be caused by a food or foods you are eating? Today I'm going to fill you in on something that has been an increasing problem amongst our population: that of food allergies or intolerances.

Any time you add something to your body that disagrees with it, it sets up the stress reaction. A sobering statistic is that there are estimated 15 million people in the United States suffering from food allergies. The yearly cost to treating just children is $25 billion. Even more sobering is that when blood from blood banks are tested, up to 60% of the donors show some intolerance to gluten and its fragments, meaning that the majority of people should be avoiding major grains such as wheat and corn. That means that an even larger percentage, potentially 200 million more cases, of untreated/ unaccounted for food allergies. This physical stress on the body contributes to the cumulative effect of all the stresses, mental, emotional, spiritual and physical you've already discovered. Add to this the degradation of our food supply, it should come as no surprise that we as a nation are not doing well compared to other nations with regards to longevity and health.

To help you understand why we have allergies or intolerances, I'll first describe what a healthy non-allergic body does after it eats food then describe what happens when someone is allergic. Then to help you discover if this is a problem for you, two at home methods that will help you determine if it is a problem. Last, the ways the Diamond Method protocol might be used to clear the food allergy from your body. The reason we'd want to do that rather than just avoid the offending food is that it limits our nutritional choices, it can create mouth boredom, and, after all, eating is a social function we do with others.

What is involved in healthy digestion?

When we eat anything there is a series a complex physical and chemical processes that ensue to make that food useful to our body. The purpose of eating is to fuel, bring energy to your cells, and to rebuild the cells broken down from normal wear and tear and injury.

You know that you have to put it in your mouth and chew. But in order to break down the food, we have a series of enzymes, called amylase, lipase and protease, which breakdown the carbohydrates, the fats, and the proteins in your food, respectively. The digestive process starts in the mouth with amylase in the saliva, breaking down the starches into sugar right away. As our food arrives in the stomach, concentrated hydrochloric acid breaks down the food even further as our stomach churns then it adds the protein and fat enzymes. This mushy mass called chyme then continues into the small intestine where a series of processes happen.

In an ideal world, proteins would be broken down completely into amino acids, carbohydrates into simple sugars, and fats into fatty acids before they enter the blood stream. These items are called macronutrients because they are the major constituents of food. There are other substances in food, that includes vitamins, minerals, non-digestible fiber, and important phytonutrients such as lycopene found in tomatoes and watermelon, all of which are healthy. These are the micronutrients (and fiber), which are in foods in relatively small quantities.

Anything that doesn't fall into the category of nutritious or healthful is filtered out by the liver and exits the body. This includes artificial sweeteners, coloring, flavors, pesticides, genetically modified food, trans fats, and any medications. Note: hormones such as thyroid or testosterone are not included in this list. Those are natural and are used by the body.

However, for most people, the standard American diet, also known as SAD for obvious reasons, has food in it that inflames (deep fried in vegetable oil, creating the inflaming trans-fats, many other inflaming foods such as crackers, frozen French fries, artificial colors, flavors, ingredients, colors, and preservatives) and causes the intestines to become swollen and permeable from micro-tears. This leads to serious health issues, as you'll see in the next sections.

What is it in the food that causes allergies?

Did you know that allergies are usually based on the protein found in the food, such as in a true milk allergy? Intolerances are caused by foods that are problematic but do not stimulate the allergic response, such as lactose in milk. It causes discomfort because of the inability for your body to break it down. You are missing an important enzyme called lactase that breaks down and transforms the lactose to something your body can use.

Common allergies are those to dairy, grains, soy, nuts, eggs, fish, seafood and to some foods containing stimulants such as caffeine and other alkaloids such as found in chocolate and tea, and even sugar.

If we were able to fully digest our foods before they entered our bloodstream, there would be no allergies to proteins in foods because they'd be broken down into individual amino acids, which are the building blocks of proteins, and these don't cause such problems. Where the trouble comes physically is that our intestines are "leaky". That means that due to some condition in the lining of our intestines, between the villi, the little finger like projections in the intestines, cracks or openings occur to the intestinal wall, allowing particles of food into the bloodstream. Our immune system reacts to that as a foreign particle and starts an inflammation cycle. This is called "leaky gut" syndrome.

Allergies can cause our bodies to exhibit a variety of symptoms and yield unexpected results.

Allergies manifest themselves in different ways in different people. Outside of the obvious symptoms of hives or skin rashes or difficulty in breathing, an allergy or intolerance may manifest itself in a huge variety of ways. Some people bloat up with water, which is the body's way of trying to dilute the irritant. Some people get foggy headed or irritable, showing that brain chemistry is affected for them. Others will get listless and tired, have some apparent phobias, show obsessive behavior, or be depressed. There can be bowel problems like IBS, stomach problems like gastric distress, and or joint inflammation. It isn't any one thing.

It occurs because polypeptides or even full-fledged proteins enter our body through the leaks in our intestines. Our body interprets these as invaders because they don't belong there. Your immune system starts making antibodies to get rid of the invading proteins/or sequence of amino acids. If your body has proteins with this same sequence of amino acids, it will start attacking itself. Common areas that are attacked are the thyroid, adrenal glands, liver, skin, joints, and bowels. These are the areas where many autoimmune diseases exhibit.

You'll even get doctors telling patients that their immune system is over active. It isn't. It's that your digestive system let the wrong guys into your blood stream activating your immune system in the first place. It is doing its job and needs to keep doing its job. The solution is first to heal the gut and to eliminate the foods causing you trouble. For the most part, following the guidelines in Chapter 9 will go a long way to eliminating inflammation. The next step is to move to a grain free "paleo" style diet, which has helped many people overcome their autoimmune issues.

My own personal story with allergies started in my late thirties and early forties. I was diagnosed with hypertension even though I was very lean, exercised daily and ate right. It turns out this was caused by a gluten allergy. After giving up gluten containing foods; sleep, digestion, and energy levels improved and my blood pressure dropped from 180/110 to 110/70 without any medication.

That wasn't the end of the story however. After menopause, I also developed a debilitating arthritis where my joints were all swollen, some severely, and the bones were starting to deform. X-rays of my hands showed bone deformation and spurs on the knuckles. After eliminating rheumatoid and osteoarthritis with a rheumatologist, inflammatory arthritis seemed to be the only choice.

As for the arthritis, after following the prescription for discovering allergies (mentioned below), I discovered that three more grains inflamed my joints. When I dropped these three grains (corn, oats and rice) from my diet: the swelling and redness subsided and the pain disappeared. It has been five years and not a single twinge of that arthritis has shown back up (unless I become contaminated by a food additive). Further positive results included dropping 10 pounds without trying and my teeth/gums stopped accumulating plaque.

The inflammation that was going on in my body died down and I got healthier over all.

The method I used to discover these allergies or intolerances was using a food/mood/energy journal jointly with muscle testing as discussed in Chapter 3. I jotted down what I ate and how I felt throughout the day. I did this for about two weeks, and a pattern emerged. I changed up my diet and food choices often. Then experimented by dropping the offending foods from my diet. This method is very easy for you to try if you suspect you have a problem or even if you don't but have one of the conditions I named in the beginning of this chapter.

If you are adept at the muscle testing mentioned in Chapter 3, you might test every food before you eat it. I test in the store before I buy. It saves me a lot of time, money, energy and days of not feeling 100%.

What is inflammation and why is it so important for you to reduce and eliminate it?

Through years of medical research, it has now become quite clear that inflammation within the body contributes to a myriad of problems including such things as the plaque build up in the arteries and eventual heart disease. Inflammation is a response of a tissue to injury, often injury caused by invading pathogens. It is characterized by increased blood flow to the tissue causing increased temperature, redness, swelling, itching and/or pain.

Inflammation can also be caused by many personal factors such as stress, smoking, viruses, consumption of refined and/or hydrogenated (trans) fats, an imbalance of omega-6 to omega-3 fats in the diet, excess refined sugars in the diet, etc. All these things are usually associated with bad health.

Can you measure inflammation by a lab test?

Levels of inflammation in your body can be measured with what's called a CRP test (c-reactive protein). The accuracy of this test still has room for improvement, as it can vary depending on the time of day and other factors, but it is a much better indication of heart disease risk than a cholesterol test, for example. This means that elevated cholesterol levels alone don't mean you are going to suffer health problems. Accompanied by inflammation, the problems have arrived.

So how does inflammation and food allergies relate to one another?

Food allergies are an extremely common affliction in both children and adults. Let's say you had a mild allergy to milk. Allergic reactions are actually caused by our bodies attempting to neutralize the foreign substance through antibodies. It doesn't kill you or endanger your life. Your body works overtime to expel the effects, so your liver gets tired, your body's immune system is taxed, your adrenal glands will get fatigued, and your intestines may even become inflamed. In this state of high alert, known as the sympathetic state, your body doesn't heal, or heals very slowly. In order for good healing to take place, your adrenal glands need to be in the "off" position, so to speak.

So, as your body is getting bombarded with this offending food, let's say it's a dairy product, day in and day out, your body isn't healing right. There's a cumulative effect of the damage. One day, the plaque accumulating in your arteries, for example, just happens to clog a coronary artery and you have a heart attack.

What are the common allergens?

While any food can potentially cause an allergic reaction, only eight foods account for 90 percent of all food allergy reactions: cow's milk, eggs, peanuts, tree nuts (for example, walnuts, pecans, almonds, and cashews), fish, shellfish, soy, corn and wheat. Because the body is reacting to something that is otherwise harmless, this type of allergic reaction is often called a hypersensitivity reaction.

An example of a food intolerance is lactose intolerance, which is due to the lack of enough of the enzyme, called lactase, to digest this milk sugar. It will cause bloating and discomfort in the intestinal tract because bacteria instead of you will digest it and produce gases.

Diagnosing food allergies is extremely difficult because most allergy tests are done on the skin surface, while food is ingested. Only some of the foods can be determined by skin tests. Even blood tests such as the celiac sprue test, which tests for gluten intolerance, can be erroneous. New research shows that the celiac sprue only tests one type of gluten intolerance and more sophisticated tests are being developed to diagnose the other types. One local clinic reports that up to 60% of the patients coming in with an apparent allergic issue have intolerances to one or more grains, mainly due to the processing modern foods undergo.

Furthermore, a single sensitivity or food allergy can cause

hypersensitivity to other related foods because the immune system is being taxed. Removing the main sensitivity can allow the immune system to recover and the secondary food will no longer be a problem. Thus, the problem is often more complex than just avoiding all the foods that cause sensitivity. Blanket elimination of food groups is really not desired as it cuts down on the variety of food (causing mouth boredom) as well as cut down on the ways we may get nourishing nutrients.

How do you determine whether you have a food allergy without a healer or doctor?

Unless you are very confident with muscle testing, the best way to determine food allergies is by doing an elimination test, where a group of foods are left off for a week to see if symptoms clear. Then foods are reintroduced and a diary kept for determining which foods are causing the inflammation. There is a great deal of information on the Internet and in libraries on "elimination diets" if you suspect you might have an allergy. It is also highly advised to find a good doctor that will work with you to help you navigate this difficult area of health.

You can try a test elimination with several foods at a time and then add them back one at a time to see if it causes a reaction. It is slow but it is also sure.

Without a healer, you can do your own muscle test by following the instructions in Chapter 3. Pick up a food and ask your body, is this food at least 70% healthy for me? I also ask, is this food going to harm my gut? Is this food going to harm my thyroid? Is this food going to cause any inflammation? If the answer is yes to any of the last 3 questions, I don't eat it.

Are the effects caused by allergies or intolerances reversible?

Most are. It can be done slowly using good nutrition after discovery of your allergy, such as the accumulation of plaque in your arteries. Once the inflammation is gone, the liver will send out the "good cholesterol" to pick up the plaque debris and carry it away opening up the arteries again. Most other problems, such as the pain and swollen joints in inflammatory arthritis will also clear, taking weeks or months as it did in my case.

Is there some way we can eat to cause fewer allergic reactions besides eliminating the offending food?

Yes, most assuredly, it is best to eliminate non-food items I mentioned earlier as much as possible. Go to organic food to avoid genetically modified foods, pesticides and added hormones to meats. Avoid artificial sweeteners, colors, flavors, trans fats, and canola oil. This will help eliminate overtaxing the liver, intestines, kidneys, adrenal glands, and thymus and help you recover.

Can allergies be "cured"?

Before I answer that, as a Scientific Healer, I know that seemingly impossible outcomes can be achieved. I've seen many transformations in situations for which conventional medicine has no answer. So, can outcomes be changed here? Emphatically yes, as I've seen them happen and experienced them myself.

Did you know that a person in a coma doesn't seem to exhibit allergies? Some doctors have said this. We must to be conscious and aware to have this allergic response to certain foods. I am not sure I'd entirely agree as some people have been accidentally poisoned by the wrong food disguised in other food; they still react. But this may be the reaction of the body to the energy of the offending food.

But this observation does give us cause to think that there is something going on emotionally or spiritually when it comes to food allergies and intolerances. In fact, my own blood tests show me allergic to only four foods, with only a mild intolerance to grains. These four foods are green beans, cinnamon, almonds and mustard. However, when I eat rice for a few days in a row, my joints inflame so much that I can't use my fingers. This speaks to an energetic allergy rather than a physical allergy.

There exists energetic clearing techniques, which you'll learn about later.

The energetic causes for allergies boil down to a few factors: DNA and family DNA, past lives, and physical problems caused by stress. There are other factors, but these are outside of the scope of what we're covering here.

Whether you ascribe to or believe in past lives, this model seems to work when it comes to clearing food allergies. In looking for the cause, I check if the origin of the food allergy came from an event in a past life. I found this is often the case and I will seek to define which life then set out to remove the influencing energetic factor.

In order to see whether clearing allergies from a past life affected them, I went to a colleague's (MD) office and used her allergy-testing machine. We tested a client, Brenda, and she registered allergic to a soft cheese, such as ricotta or cottage cheese. I found that in three previous lives, this was an issue. As I removed the cause energetically, I felt a resistance in my fingers, as if I were uprooting a weed. I pulled it free. When we retested Brenda after a few minutes, her body no longer registered as allergic to this particular dairy product. This was a major factor in her allergy. Often this is not enough. We tested Brenda again a few days later, and the response on the machine showed an allergy to soft cheese again. There are still more factors to overcome.

Isn't there more to allergies than past lives?

To complete the process of clearing allergies, I also check for DNA issues that may be inherited from one or both parents and reset the DNA program energetically so it is no longer a problem. This is done via a simple energetic process by which the "faulty" information is replaced by healthy information from your healthy energetic blueprint. I'd like to remind you that we all carry a healthy energetic blueprint around and that activating it helps remove the allergy stemming from inheriting it. There's a minor piece to this and that is we all come from a biological or spiritual tribe. We have similar beliefs. Often this group thinking moves into an allergic reaction to a food. To further clear this allergy, I energetically disconnect you from this family thought process for this one issue.

There are also concepts that are faulty in current times. For example, in one culture, tomatoes were forbidden because several varieties of them were poisonous. This was therefore a protective device. In our markets, we don't have any poisonous tomatoes, so banishing them based on this old thinking is not serving us any more. I remove the energy of these kinds of thoughts from affecting you.

Lastly, there are physical issues around allergies that include the small intestine, the large intestine, the liver, the thymus, the adrenal glands, the brain, and the thyroid. The kidneys may also be involved. I also check for areas of inflammation that may accompany these allergies. In all these cases, the physical parts of you that are affected are brought up to full energy and healed using your perfect energetic blueprint.

Since there is some sort of inertia in our faulty thinking and health patterns that are causing the allergy, I will go back and double check a client a week or two later to make sure the new programming holds and they are not going to react violently to a food. I give them a boost and search for more causes if there is some backsliding. Since allergies can be dangerous, this kind of clearing is a topic of ongoing research and future plans include intermittent testing on an allergy machine until all causes have been found and eliminated.

Often a more non-invasive procedure such as NAET is helpful to overcome allergies. NAET is an energetic process that reprograms your nervous system to stop reacting to the food or environmental factor any longer. A prudent doctor will also administer a comprehensive blood test before and after. Many anaphylactic reactions to peanuts, seafood and other problematic allergens have been mitigated or eliminated by this technique. It is powerful and it does work.

Energetically clearing allergies works, but the responsible healer would not give you the go ahead without having you tested physically. One healer gave this advice to a psychiatric patient. She was horribly allergic to milk, causing her to have psychotic and suicidal episodes. That healer said the allergy was clear but obviously it was only momentary as when the patient ingested milk again, she went into a psychotic episode. Clearing a lifetime (or lifetimes) of a food issue takes more than one sitting and it takes the coordination of your healer with your doctor to make sure you come to no harm and are clear once and for all of this issue.

You've just read all about allergies, how they manifest, how you can discover them, how you can get relief from their symptoms, and how you can clear them from your body. Seek out a Scientific Healer to get more help if you are stuck.

Photo: Carolina Biological Supply Company, 2012

10. Self-care is the foundation of self-love

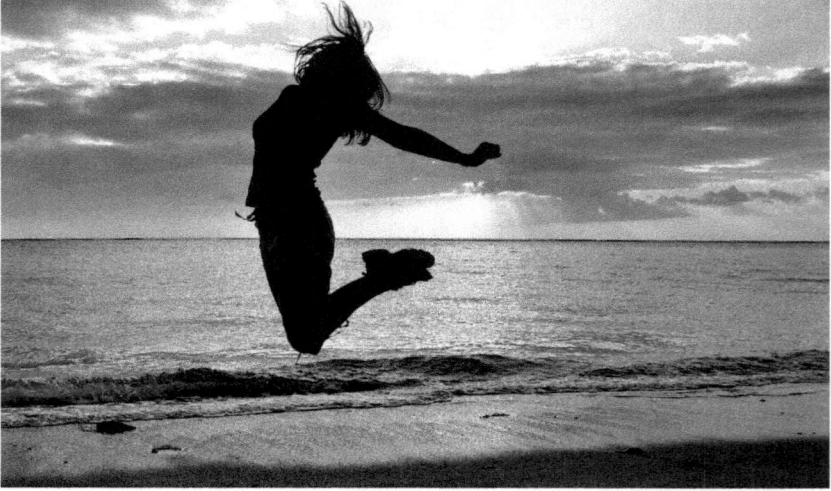

"Behind every stressful thought is the desire for things to be other than they are."
Toni Bernhard

One important factor that supports your resiliency is making sure your body is being well nourished and rested. It will give you the physical and mental strength and stamina to go through any challenge when needed. By caring for yourself, you are telling your body that you believe you are valuable. When you do this, it responds positively to your care. Self-love is the basis for great relationships, a great career, abundance, and vibrant health.

There are four important factors in self-care: first is cleaning up the diet and environment, second is nourishing food on the right schedule, the third is resting, and the forth is exercise. All those are common sense. The first, cleaning up the diet, is probably the most profound as the current state of the food supply in the United States is not to be taken at face value. What appears to be normal healthy food is in actuality unhealthy food in disguise. If you look at the upturn in the number of problems including obesity, mental illness, occurrence of diabetes, autism, cancer, etc. The frequency of cases can be directly correlated to the adulteration of our food supply, the toxins, the genetic modifications, the synthetic ingredients, and artificial sweeteners.

Let's start examining each component of self care starting with cleaning up your diet.

Cleaning up your body is a key step to vitality

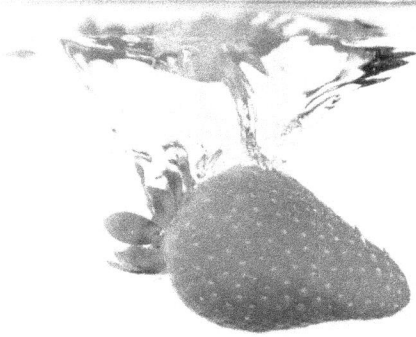

Cleaning up your body: an important step to better health. Your body has a system of purification organs including the liver, kidneys, skin, spleen, and the lymph system. One of the most important of these that I find depleted in many clients is the liver. As soon as you start overloading the body with things that are not nourishing, not rebuilding or supplying energy to the body, the liver goes into over drive as do your adrenal glands. This includes the bulk of medications. Anything that goes "against the grain" will cause your adrenal glands to fire.

As mentioned, your liver is a marvel of biological function. It has many primary functions, which are all necessary for health and survival. These include detoxification, protein synthesis, production of digestive juices, glycogen storage, breakdown of "tired" red blood cells, regulating the cholesterol in your body, and plays a primary role in metabolism. As a note, your capacity for your liver to handle toxins may vary from the average person. Some of you are not as capable of handling a heavy toxic load, such as those things mentioned later in this chapter. Why not give your body a break and eat "cleanly" as much as possible

When you overtax the liver with toxins and non-food substances, it can't perform the functions it is supposed to, like supplying us with energy, carrying the "bad" cholesterol out of the system, produce the good cholesterol, and rid our system of the "debris".

Don't go about randomly tossing out foods or whole food groups unless you are allergic to them or there is scientific evidence showing it is dangerous, unhealthy, cancerous or tumor fodder. You might also have to leave some of your favorite "vices" behind and regard food as nourishing rather than recreational in order to get healthy again. You might not think this is so much fun, but it actually is because you'll feel so much better and hardly go to the doctor, just for checkups. Fun will have a whole new meaning.

Each topic briefly covered in this chapter could occupy a whole chapter or even book. Suffice it to say, if some of these "baddies" are not proven yet, there is a large body of scientific and anecdotal evidence against each one. There are also large agri- and chemical-lobbies that are keeping these items in the food supplies. So, take it all in stride. Choose what you'd like to do for yourself. Making you aware of them will help you start to choose better options.

The first step to cleaning and detoxing your body is plenty of fresh/ clean water.

Water is of utmost importance to your health

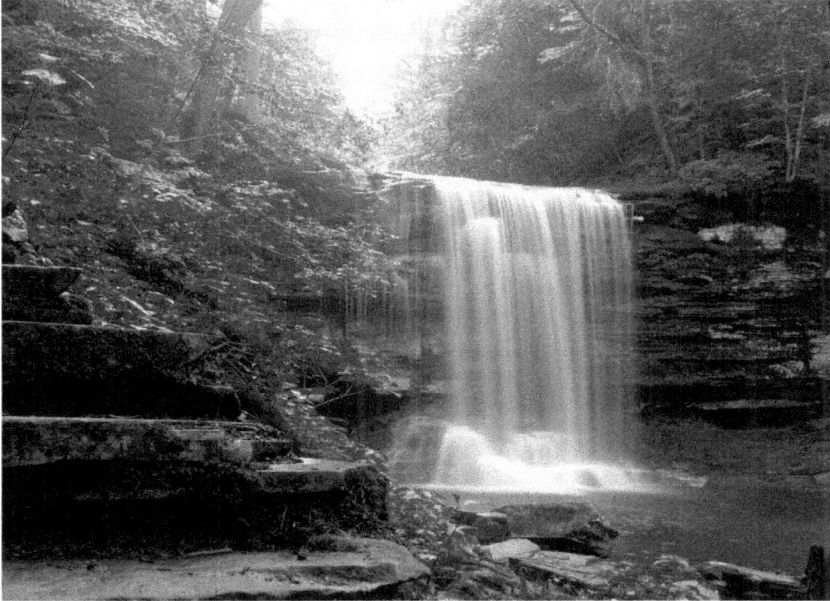

Water is one of the most forgotten "cures" to many problems. It is especially essential for detoxing your body. Drinking a healthy amount of water is vital to your health. You would never imagine that just by adding this simple habit, you would become healthier! Let's look at the role of water in your body.

We are 2/3 water!

Your body is about 67% (2/3) water, with the tissues and organs containing the larger percentages:

Muscle consists of 75% water

Brain consists of 90% water

Bone consists of 22% water

Blood consists of 83% water

The functions of water in your body are vital. The water:

Transports nutrients and oxygen into cells

Moisturizes the air in lungs

Helps with metabolism

Protects your vital organs

Helps your organs to absorb nutrients better

Regulates body temperature

Detoxifies
Protects and moisturizes our joints
Reduces the toxic load in your body
Helps your brain function, think clearly (it's 90% water!)
Maintains chemical balance

Every cell in your body needs water from head to toe. That is why it is so important to drink enough fluid, especially plain water (to give your liver a break). Take for example, without enough water, your brain won't function well and you will likely get a headache or migraine. Hence, next time, if you feel fatigue and headache, it may be the sign of dehydration.

Effects of Dehydration:

It is probably surprising to you that all these may be a result of simple dehydration.
Tiredness
Migraine
Constipation
Muscle cramps
Irregular blood pressure
Kidney problems
Dry skin
20% dehydrated – Risk of death

Symptoms of Dehydration

While those effects are the results, you may not yet be suffering any of them. If you have the following, added water will definitely relieve symptoms:
- Dark Urine – Dark Yellow or Orange in Color: Urine is generally pale yellow to clear when you have sufficient water intake. Dark color or strong smell indicates that you need to drink more water.
- Dry Skin: Skin is the largest body organ and requires its share of water.
- Thirst: Thirst is the most obvious sign that you're already dehydrated. It is always a good practice to drink more water when you are not thirsty; don't wait until you're thirsty.

- Hunger: Most people mistake hunger as an indication to eat more, whereas in actual fact, you may be dehydrated. So before you have your meal, grab a glass of water.
- Fatigue: Water gives you a boost in energy.

How much water should you drink a day to avoid dehydration and stay healthy?

There is no clear cut answer as to how much water to drink per day, because it depends upon a number of factors like your health condition, your activity status, the climatic conditions, physical size, your weight, your environment, etc. You lose quite a lot of water through sweating, exhaling and urinating. In hot weather, you tend to lose more water through sweating. In cold conditions, you tend to urinate more. In the event of sickness like flu and diarrhea, you tend to lose fluid. When you weigh more, your body needs more fluid for muscles, organs, bones etc.

I'm sure you've heard it said that you should drink 8 glasses of water a day (unfortunately there are a lot of people that don't!). At 8 ounces per glass, this is approximately half a gallon or two liters of water a day. Is drinking 8 glasses of water enough? A more accurate estimation is to drink at least half your body weight (in pounds) in ounces of water. If it is hot or you sweat a lot drink more.

This means if you weigh 160 lbs, this is 80 ounces, a bit more than the 64 ounces provided by the 8 glasses a day recommendation.

Water is helpful for weight loss for two reasons:

Water flushes the toxins out of the body, so your body doesn't store them away in your fat cells (which is where they tend to be stored to keep them out of your bloodstream). It helps the liver do its job of detoxifying so the excess fat storage is no longer necessary for toxin removal.

Often thirst is mistaken as hunger, more water will prevent you from eating more. You can get by on less food, because once thirst is satisfied, you no longer crave something. The satisfied thirst really curbs appetite.

Water has zero calories. Some people complain it doesn't taste good. Look around for different combinations of minerals in drinking water. Some will taste better than others for you. Add lemon or lime to it to give it a little oomph without a lot of sugar. Or simply get used to it: you'll find your mind so awake with it that you'll start to enjoy the flavor more.

Carbonated water is not recommended for liberal consumption. It should be straight "still" water. The excess carbonation is not good for bone density

So, as you can see, water is very beneficial to your body and you should not hesitate to drink it.

Curtail Alcohol Consumption
This is an obvious one for the effect alcohol has on the liver and brain. Of course, books and books have been written on the topic. We know it taxes the liver and that liver disease can be the result of overindulgence of alcohol. It also hinders brain function, which is required if your body is to stay healthy, and may even kill brain neurons.

It is said that a small glass of red wine will help prevent strokes and heart attacks. That doesn't mean half a bottle like I've seen some people do, telling me that it is "healthy". Alcohol is metabolized but at the expense of our liver. You are trying to get your liver (and brain) to function optimally to allow you to become vibrant and alive. Alcohol makes that task more difficult than it needs to be. Thus, the prudent course of action is to curtail it.

Alcohol should be stopped temporarily in the weeks following a brain healing. In general, I've seen the brain go back to its pre-healed state once alcohol is consumed. This means all the work that was done to improve the brain is wiped out.

Stop Smoking

Smoking is one of the most insidious habits. It is really tough to quit. My brother-in-law had three heart attacks by age 52. He managed to lose 90 lbs (he is very tall) but still can't get rid of the cigarettes despite trying to quit several times. Do whatever you can to quit and don't take it lightly.

Those e-cigarettes are a great help. A number of people have been able to stop smoking using these. Brandon tried several times to quit. In a period of two weeks, with an e-cigarette he was able to quit and cut down on his e-cigarette use without an increase in appetite or eating more.

It is well known that cigarettes put poison in our bodies, but also those around us. Even after we've finished the cigarette, the chemicals that sit on our clothing and linger on our furniture is still coming into our lungs. It ages us very quickly, we get wrinkled, it depletes our nutrients, it depletes our lung capacity. I've lost important people in my life that were younger than I am now from smoking. Please don't be one of those too.

Curtail sugar consumption

Too much sugar puts undue stress on your body. It actually burns up the inside of your blood vessels if the concentration in your bloodstream is too high. This in itself will raise inflammation to very high levels causing a cascade of bad health effects. Even though it qualifies as "food", it is something that needs to be curtailed or eliminated. Get your sweets from natural foods, like whole fresh fruits. Keep dried fruit to a minimum.

Cleaning up your diet is important

The best things to avoid taking in or using are things that aren't food and water. You might think I'm going to tell you that it's artificial colors and preservatives, and you'd be partially right. There are a few surprising things as well. Some of these are even advertised as healthy or harmless, but judging by the reactions of the people I tell about these items and their general improvement in health after avoiding them, it is worth testing.

So here are the obvious things to avoid:
  Artificial flavors

Artificial colors
Nitrates and Nitrites
Preservatives, such as BHA, BHT, etc.
Artificial Sweeteners, aspartame, sucralose, neotame, acesulfame potassium, and saccharine, (see if stevia works for you)
Drugs
Maltodextrin
High fructose corn syrup
Canola oil
GMO foods

Eliminate MSG

Flavor enhancers have msg or monosodium glutamate in them. MSG itself is addicting to many people. It is an excitotoxin. It has infiltrated practically all packaged food. It takes some people three days to recover from an accidental dose (usually at restaurants, if it tastes too good, there's probably a reason. The reason is msg.)

The packages containing msg also name it with other names so we don't really realize that we are getting msg:
Monosodium Glutamate
Hydrolyzed Vegetable Protein
Hydrolyzed Protein
Hydrolyzed Plant Protein
Plant Protein Extract
Sodium Caseinate
Calcium Caseinate
Yeast Extract
Textured Protein (Including TVP)
Autolyzed Yeast
Hydrolyzed Oat Flour
Corn Oil
Plus many more

Processed food

A recent disturbing statistic is that 90% of all purchased food is processed. This means that all those chemicals named above and msg in its many forms is pumped into our bodies and our livers are working overtime trying to eliminate these things from our bodies.

Trans-Fatty Acids and Hydrogenated Fat

You'll want to avoid -- **in fact eliminate altogether** – your consumption of trans-fatty acids. A U.S. government panel of scientists determined that man-made trans fats are unsafe at any level.

This man-made fat is produced by heating polyunsaturated vegetable oil until it breaks down chemically into a gray goo. To make it look better, for instance like butter, it is bleached and tinted yellow, then chemical flavor enhancers added to make it taste like butter. It's been said it is one step away from being plastic. The purpose of heating up the oil is to make it solid and stable. It can be pressed into bars and sold as a butter substitute. This fat is not found in nature, you can't extract it from a plant. It does not contain cholesterol as fatty meats and eggs do, but the consequences are much worse. After companies started pushing this relatively cheap source of fat as the way to get butter without the "problems" butter caused, it was discovered that, in actuality, margarines caused a worse buildup of plaque in arteries than butter ever did. It is a non-food stuff that disrupts liver function amongst other things.

Margarines and packaged food with hydrogenated oils and fats are all best to be avoided. Places you'll find trans fatty acids are in packaged crackers like wheat thins, deep fried foods like potato chips, mac and cheese, doughnuts and corn chips, margarines and other veggie spreads made from liquid oils but solidified by thermal degradation. Be most wary of this fat.

Rather, opt for butter, healthy oils, lemon juice, herbs, and spices to add flavor, and get rid of all added salts and fats. LESS SALT IS ALSO GOOD FOR YOU. It doesn't affect cholesterol levels but it will affect blood pressure. Limit your sodium intake to 2400 milligrams a day

Some experts have labeled this fat the largest mistake in food history. That may be closer to the truth than anyone could possibly guess.

The New Cholesterol Lowering Margarines

The FDA has approved two sterol-containing margarines as "foods". Benecol contains sterol from pine tree wood pulp ("food"?) and that in Take Control is derived from soybean oil. Sterols resemble cholesterol chemically. The stanol esters in Benecol are produced from sterols by hydrogenation and esterification with unsaturated fatty acids. The margarines also still contain partially hydrogenated other materials. There is short term evidence that these are "safe" and do slightly reduce cholesterol. The maximum effective dosage is about a tablespoon and a half of margarine. There are no long-term studies.

However, there have been some downsides to these compounds as can be expected. Serum concentrations of plant sterols have been associated with premature coronary disease. Patients with inherited sitosterolemia, a lipid metabolic disorder, are known to develop xanthomas, a disfiguring deposit of yellow cholesterol under the skin, and premature ischemic heart disease. Plant sterols behave estrogenically, meaning they can cause endocrine problems; in animals these sterols contribute to sexual inversion (a reversal of gender traits). Both margarines may decrease plasma concentrations of antioxidants and beta-carotene. Supplementation of these nutrients needs to be increased. Both margarines cost about 5 times that of ordinary margarine.

Why You Should Avoid Margarine, Shortening and Spreads

Aside from the trans-fats and plant sterols that we already discussed, margarines contain a number of other harmful substances including:
1. **Free radicals:** Free radicals and other toxic breakdown products are the result of high temperature industrial processing of vegetable oils. They are known to contribute to health problems, including cancer and heart disease.
2. **Synthetic vitamins:** Synthetic vitamin A and other vitamins are added to margarine and spreads. These often have an opposite (and detrimental) effect compared to the natural vitamins in butter.

3. **Emulsifiers and preservatives:** Numerous additives of questionable safety are added to margarines and spreads. Most vegetable shortening is stabilized with preservatives like BHT.

4. **Hexane and other solvents:** used in the extraction process. These industrial chemicals can have toxic effects. Many are carcinogenic.

5. **Bleach:** The natural color of partially hydrogenated vegetable oil is grey, which is not so appetizing. Manufacturers first bleach it to make it white then add yellow dyes to make it resemble butter.

6. **Artificial flavors**: These help mask the terrible taste and odor of partially hydrogenated oils, and provide a fake butter taste.

7. **Mono- and di-glycerides:** These contain trans fats that manufacturers do not have to list on the label. They are used in high amounts in so-called "low-trans" spreads.

8. **Soy protein isolate:** This highly processed powder is added to "low-trans" spreads to give them body. It can contribute to thyroid dysfunction, digestive disorders and many other health problems, which is mentioned in a later section.

What is a Canola?

Canola oil is being pushed as a healthy fat because it has a lot of monounsaturated fat, but may be as much a fiasco as margarine and trans fats were. To answer the question, what is a canola: There is no such plant as a canola plant. The "can" stands for Canada, and "ola" for oil.

Canola oil is actually oil pressed from rapeseed, which is a plant from the mustard seed family. In its original state, it is toxic due to concentrations of **erucic acid**. In the late 1970s, Canadian plant breeders were able to create a variety of rapeseed that produced a mono-unsaturated oil, which was much lower in erucic acid, and is probably not much of a problem except to the very sensitive. A worse problem is that during processing, high heat is used causing the oils to break down to trans-fats. Levels up to 4.6% trans-fat have been measured in these oils!

Read the labels of all food products and avoid this oil. You might also find the taste (and odor) much like motor oil because it is broken down in the heating process, it's not nearly as tasty as real food oils such as olive oil, almond oil, sesame oil, all of which add wonderful flavors to food as well as being superb for health. Most doctors are not aware of this problem (much like the margarine fiasco). As mentioned before, they are also inundated with the same misinformation as the rest of us.

Soy is unhealthy!
Increasing levels of soy intake is emphatically not recommend, particularly unfermented soy, in your diet and here's why. Soy has been implicated as problematic for many people, especially for those with thyroid issues. Did you know the number one prescribed medicine in 2013 is thyroid hormone?

You might also find anything made with soy protein full of weird ingredients that you can't pronounce or spell! Often, the food manufacturers make up for the lack of flavor by adding too much salt and too much fat. It defeats the purpose, doesn't it? Ever had a protein bar made with soy protein? Some taste like chocolate covered sawdust.

Vegetarians might consider eating fish or eggs for protein: sorry, but soy is just not a healthy choice at all.

Furthermore, most non-organic soy in the USA is genetically modified. It is also in virtually every packaged food item, either as oil, lecithin, or protein. Be on the lookout for it.

Avoid White Food

White food, such as white flour and white sugar, is food that has been stripped of the nutritional value/fiber and repackaged. It isn't done for flavor; it is done because it lasts longer on the shelves. However, these are devoid of most nutrition and add empty calories to our diet. The other problem with white food is that it lacks fiber and the germ where the oils and nutrients are. The result is that it becomes easy to digest and is sent quickly into our bloodstream where it shoots our blood sugar levels up way too quickly. Shortly after that, it is just as quickly swept out of the bloodstream by insulin.

Consumption of refined white food is associated with many health problems particularly because of the spiking of blood sugar then depletion of energy in our system. New research shows that wildly swinging blood sugar levels actually increases blood lipid levels. Decreasing intake of these high glycemic foods, i.e., ones that are digested and moved into the bloodstream quickly, actually increases your good cholesterol levels.

Why Butter is Better

1. **Vitamins:** Butter is a rich source of easily absorbed vitamin A and also contains all the other fat-soluble vitamins (D, E and K2), which are often lacking in the modern industrial diet.
2. **Minerals:** Butter is rich in important trace minerals, including manganese, chromium, zinc, copper and selenium (a powerful antioxidant). Butter provides more selenium per gram than wheat germ or herring. Butter is also an excellent source of iodine.
3. **Fatty Acids:** Butter provides appreciable amounts of short- and medium-chain fatty acids, which support immune function, boost metabolism and have anti-microbial properties; that is, they fight against pathogenic microorganisms in the intestinal tract. Butter also provides the perfect balance of omega-3 and omega-6 fats. Arachidonic acid in butter is important for brain function, skin health and prostaglandin balance. Butter contains about 100 different fatty acids, many of which are beneficial but not found in other foods such as conjugated linoleic acid, or CLA, and glycospingolipids, GSL. CLA gives excellent protection against cancer and also helps your body build muscle rather than store fat. GSLs are a special category of fatty acids that protect against gastrointestinal infections, especially in the very young and the elderly.
4. **Cholesterol**: Despite all of the misinformation you may

have heard, cholesterol is needed to maintain intestinal health and for brain and nervous system development in the young.

5. **Wulzen Factor:** A hormone-like substance that prevents arthritis and joint stiffness, ensuring that calcium in your body is put into your bones rather than your joints and other tissues. The Wulzen factor is present only in raw butter and cream; it is destroyed by pasteurization.

Butter helps in the following conditions:

1. **Heart Disease:** Butter contains many nutrients that protect against heart disease including vitamins A, D, K2, and E, lecithin, iodine and selenium. A Medical Research Council survey showed that men eating butter ran half the risk of developing heart disease as those using margarine (Nutrition Week 3/22/91, 21:12).

2. **Cancer:** The short- and medium-chain fatty acids in butter have strong anti-tumor effects. Conjugated linoleic acid (CLA) in butter from grass-fed cows also gives excellent protection against cancer.

3. **Arthritis:** The Wulzen or "anti-stiffness" factor in raw butter and also Vitamin K2 in grass-fed butter, protect against calcification of the joints as well as hardening of the arteries, cataracts and calcification of the pineal gland. Calves fed pasteurized milk or skim milk develop joint stiffness and do not thrive.

4. **Osteoporosis:** Vitamins A, D and K2 in butter are essential for the proper absorption of calcium and phosphorus and hence necessary for strong bones and teeth.

5. **Thyroid Health:** Butter is a good source of iodine, in a highly absorbable form. Butter consumption prevents goiter in mountainous areas where seafood is not available. In addition, vitamin A in butter is essential for proper functioning of the thyroid gland.

6. **Digestion:** Glycospingolipids in butterfat protect against gastrointestinal infection, especially in the very young and the elderly.

7. **Growth & Development:** Many factors in the butter ensure optimal growth of children, especially iodine and

vitamins A, D and K2. Low-fat diets have been linked to failure to thrive in children -- yet low-fat diets are often recommended for youngsters!

8. **Asthma:** Saturated fats in butter are critical to lung function and protect against asthma

9. **Overweight**: CLA and short- and medium-chain fatty acids in butter help control weight gain.

10. **Fertility**: Many nutrients contained in butter are needed for fertility and normal reproduction.

It is clear that natural substances are far superior to any man made substance. If you can find it, use grass fed organic and, better, raw unpasteurized butter from a reliable source. It will have a very healthy fatty acid content. Your taste buds will definitely thank you too.

Eat Organic Where Possible

If you are a non-believer thinking that organic food is just expensive food, there are actually several valid and important reasons for promoting organic food. It has to do not only with our internal health, but also our external environment. Sure, they tend to be a little more expensive, but if we demand them in stores, the prices do drop. We vote with our wallets. Wal-Mart, for example, noticed a higher demand for organics and contracted with organic farmers for organic dairy products, many of which are only slightly higher priced. Similarly, other food chains such as Ralph's (a Kroger store) has adopted its own organic brands. Some people might not be able afford these. But really, our lives and health depend on getting good food. It is definitely a lot cheaper to not need doctors, medications, and have very few sick days. In the long run, it is worth it. You have to decide for yourself if you want to go this route. At least move towards organic dairy products and free-range eggs, many of which are about the same cost as conventional products.

First, organic food is produced without pesticides. The pesticides are washed into the water supply when it rains or the crops are watered. It affects our environment, and other plants and animals are poisoned with it. One example of where this was disastrous was DDT. Our foul were dying off because the eggshells were decalcified and not lasting through incubation. Ingesting pesticides on our produce overworks our liver so it can't do other functions. They may be poisonous to us: long-term effects are not yet known.

At the very least, start substituting produce with the highest pesticide residues for those that are less contaminated. The lists below should help with that. First, produce with the lowest pesticide residues are listed. Then comes a table with produce with the highest pesticide residues next to some better substitutions with lower residue levels. At least, if not organic, at least better for you and your family.

Here are the foods with the lowest pesticide residues:
Avocados
Corn
Onions
Sweet Potatoes
Cauliflower
Brussels Sprouts
Grapes (US, Mexico)
Bananas
Plums
Green Onions
Watermelon
Broccoli

Table 10-1 Table of Pesticide-Rich Foods & Substitutes

Pesticide Rich	Equivalent Nutrient Substitution
Strawberries	Blackberries, raspberries, blueberries, kiwi, orange, cantaloupe
Bell Peppers ...Green	Green peas, broccoli, romaine lettuce
Bell Peppers ...Red	Carrots, broccoli, Brussels sprouts, tomatoes, asparagus, romaine lettuce
Spinach	Broccoli, Brussels sprouts, asparagus, romaine lettuce
Cherries (US)	Grapefruit, blueberries, raspberries, cantaloupe, oranges
Peaches	Nectarines, canned peaches, cantaloupe (US), tangerine, grapefruit, watermelon
Cantaloupe (Mexico)	Watermelon, cantaloupe (US)
Celery	Carrots, broccoli, radishes, romaine lettuce
Apples	Oranges, nectarines, bananas, kiwis, watermelon, tangerines
Apricots	Nectarines, cantaloupe (US), watermelon, tangerines, grapefruit
Green Beans	Green peas, broccoli, cauliflower, Brussels sprouts, asparagus
Grapes (Chile)	Grapes (US), in season
Cucumbers	Carrots, romaine lettuce, broccoli, radishes

Pears	Canned pears, canned peaches, oranges, nectarines
Winter Squash (US)	Winter squash (Honduras, Mexico), sweet potatoes (US)
Potatoes (US)	Sweet potatoes (US), carrots, winter squash (Honduras, Mexico)

Second, organic food is produced without added antibiotics. The antibiotics cause problems in themselves. Many people are allergic to them. They are estrogenic and men can experience low sperm counts and female body characteristics. Did you know that many American foods are banned in Europe due to antibiotic use? Too many added antibiotics also cause resistant strains of bacteria to thrive, many of which have become deadly. Many hospitals have these problems.

Third, organic foods are produced with natural rather than chemical fertilizers, increasing the nutrient content and flavor of our foods. Using natural fertilizers is like feeding plants health foods. They are more bug resistant, heartier and require fewer precautions against pest destruction. Besides, this makes them tastier.

Fourth, organic and free-range animals, also called sustainably farmed, are treated more humanely. Free-range chickens and their eggs aren't cooped up in dark places their whole lives. Their conditions are a great deal more sanitary, and their food superior. Cows aren't stuffed with grains, which cause stomach and intestinal distress and bacterial growth. This then requires the use of antibiotics. In addition, the animals treated more humanely are healthier for us because their flesh isn't riddled with stress hormones and undue bacteria from unsanitary conditions.

Fifth, organic or sustainably farmed food is not genetically modified. The purpose of these modifications is to make the crops impervious to herbicides so the farmers don't have to weed between the crop rows. Instead they just spray "Roundup" made by Monsanto, for example, to do the weeding for them, which means we also get that into our food supply. New studies are showing the levels of herbicidal toxins in these foods have risen to unacceptable levels.

New studies also show that if the molecule was never in our food supply in the first place, adding new ones means our bodies do not know how to deal with it. The brain doesn't signal the body to stop being hungry or the body can't process it. Laboratory rats eating GMO (genetically modified organism) foods have become sterile after 2 to 3 generations. Europe has banned GMO foods. Therefore, many U.S. foods cannot be imported into European countries. It seems outrageous that we could be rendering our own population sterile for someone's convenience.

Let me demonstrate how even a slightly modified food can be deadly. L-carnitine is necessary for the liver's ability to transport energy to the muscles. Its sister molecule D-carnitine is deadly as it stops energy transport to the muscles, including the heart, and we die ingesting it. The difference between the two is the geometric arrangement of only one bond. It has the exact same composition! That one bond change renders it deadly. This should allay any arguments about the nearness of chemical composition. Here it's identical, it's only the arrangement that's different. So, rather than risk long-term problems, the prudent choice is to not eat GMO food.

Summary and Action Plan

Try one or more of the recommendations in this chapter. The recommended order of the ideas in this chapter:
1. Drop trans fat
2. Cut down smoking and drinking
3. Cut down artificial ingredients/chemicals/colorings preservatives
4. Eat less white foods
5. Cut out GMO foods such as canola oil, soy, and non-organic corn
6. Go organic

Besides removing future toxins from the body, another great way to remove stress from your body is to help it detox the toxins you've already eaten. A big step to achieving this is drinking plenty of water: the topic of the next chapter.

Action steps from this chapter:

1. Besides the obvious lifestyle changes of cutting down on smoking and drinking, read the labels of everything in your frig, freezer and pantry. If you are so inclined (as I was), get a big trash bag and start throwing out the worst offenders. It is somehow freeing to toss the poisonous food out.

2. Afterwards, go shopping for some single or two ingredient foods. Like apples, broccoli, salmon, almonds, butter, olive oil. Try shopping at stores like Trader Joe's and Whole Foods where you can find less expensive organic foods. Whole Food's 365 Brand is usually less expensive than those found in regular chain super markets such as Kroger/QFC/Ralphs.

3. Start gearing your kitchen up to move towards healthier eating. It doesn't mean more time consuming. Healthy frozen fruit and vegetables only take a few minutes to warm up and eat. Cook in bulk and divide it down. You can get several meals from one preparation time. Freeze some for later and eat the same for a meal or two.

4. Start now, don't wait until you read the rest of the book. Eliminating chemical ingredients is a HUGE step in the right direction.

Rest is the fountain of youth

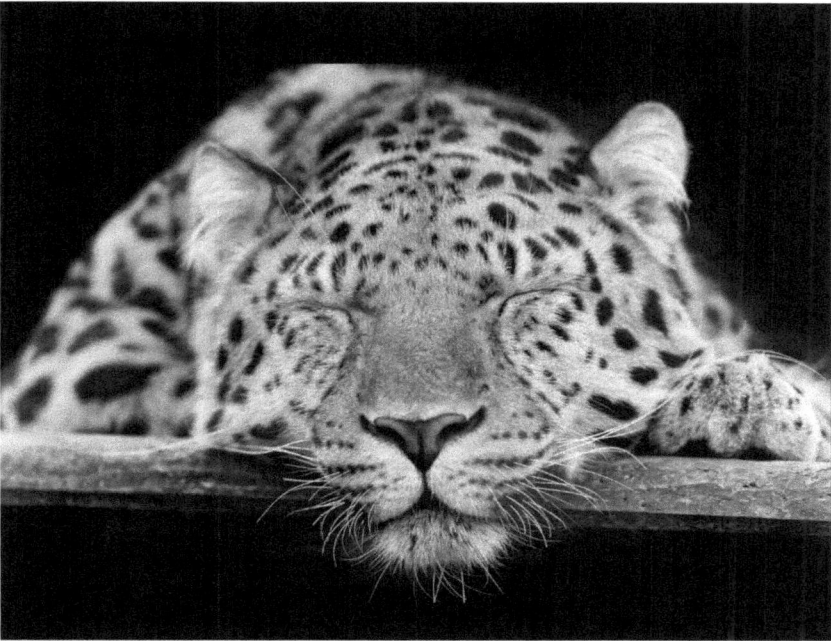

We can be doing all the right things, but we can offset a lot of the good we are doing if we do not rest well. All sorts of nasty hormones get released into our bloodstream, including cortisol. The stress hormones will increase blood pressure, raise cholesterol, make us fatter, especially around the belly, and generally make us miserable. Exercise, as covered in the next section, helps counteract the stress hormones but it can't make up for lack of sleep or rest. Barring any physical problem, you need more sleep if you:

Need an alarm clock or rely on the snooze button.

Have a hard time getting out of bed in the morning.

Feel sluggish in the afternoon.

Get sleepy in meetings, lectures, or warm rooms.

Get drowsy after heavy meals or when driving.

Need to nap to get through the day.

Fall asleep while watching TV or relaxing in the evening.

Feel the need to sleep in on weekends.

Fall asleep within five minutes of going to bed.

But getting enough sleep is very important to our overall health. If you have no other known physical issue, effects of lack of sleep or

chronic sleep deprivation include:
Fatigue, lethargy, and lack of motivation
Moodiness and irritability
Reduced creativity and problem-solving skills
Inability to cope with stress
Reduced immunity; frequent colds and infections
Concentration and memory problems
Increased cravings, hunger, and weight gain
Impaired motor skills and increased risk of accidents
Difficulty making decisions
Increased risk of diabetes, heart disease, and other health problems

Sleep Makes You Smarter

Studies show that learning is affected by lack of sleep. The best learning occurs when a person rests both before and after learning. At least 6 hours of sleep is required to show improvement in learning. Furthermore, those that slept 8 hours outperformed those that slept only 6 or 7 hours.

It is suspected that while people sleep, they form or reinforce pathways that brain cells need to perform a task. Sleep is needed for proper brain development in infants.

Several studies show that lack of sleep causes thinking processes to slow down. Lack of sleep also makes it harder to focus and pay attention. Lack of sleep can make you more easily confused. Studies also find a lack of sleep leads to faulty decision-making and more risk taking. Lack of sleep slows down your reaction time, which is particularly important for driving (and other tasks that require quick responses). When people who lack sleep are tested on a driving simulator, they perform just as poorly as people who are drunk. The bottom line is: not getting a good night's sleep not only makes us dumb, it can be dangerous!

Sleep improves mood

We have a nation of people that are taking psychotropic drugs for depression. However, a good night's sleep can put you in a better mood.

Most people report being irritable, if not downright unhappy, when they lack sleep. People who chronically suffer from a lack of sleep, are at greater risk of developing depression. One group of people who usually don't get enough sleep is mothers of newborns. Some experts think depression after childbirth (postpartum blues) is caused, in part, by a lack of sleep.

A lack of sleep puts your body under stress and that triggers the release of adrenaline, cortisol, and other stress hormones during the day. This is the start of a vicious cycle: these hormones contribute to your blood pressure not dropping during sleep, thereby increasing the risk for heart disease.

Blood levels of certain proteins such as C-reactive protein are increased through lack of sleep. C-reactive protein indicates inflammation and is associated with atherosclerosis or hardening of the arteries.

Sleep improves Muscle Growth and Metabolism

Deep sleep triggers the release of growth hormone, which boosts muscle mass and the repair of cells and tissues. This is part of the rest that athletes need to stay in top form and make sure they can perform at their best. In order to maintain a good healthy metabolism and active vibrant brain, muscle mass is required (muscle is metabolically active).

 Sleep Keeps us Healthy and Lean

During sleep, your body creates more cytokines — cellular hormones that help the immune system fight various infections. Lack of sleep can reduce the ability to fight off common infections. Research also reveals that a lack of sleep can reduce the body's response to the flu vaccine. For example, sleep-deprived volunteers given the flu vaccine produced less than half as many flu antibodies as those who were well rested and given the same vaccine.

Although lack of exercise and other factors are important contributors, the current epidemic of diabetes and obesity appears to be related, at least in part, to chronically getting inadequate sleep.

Evidence is growing that sleep is a powerful regulator of appetite, energy use, and weight control. During sleep, the body's production of the appetite suppressor *leptin* increases, and the appetite stimulant *grehlin* decreases. Studies find that the less people sleep, the more likely they are to be overweight or obese and prefer eating foods that are higher in calories and carbohydrates. People who report an average total sleep time of 5 hours a night, for example, are much more likely to become obese compared to people who sleep 7–8 hours a night.

A number of hormones released during sleep also control the body's use of energy. A distinct rise and fall of blood sugar levels during sleep appears to be linked to sleep stage. Not getting enough sleep overall or enough of each stage of sleep disrupts this pattern. One study found that, when healthy young men slept only 4 hours a night for 6 nights in a row, their insulin and blood sugar levels mimicked those seen in people who were developing diabetes. Another study found that women who slept *less than 7 hours* a night were more likely to develop diabetes over time than those who slept between 7 and 8 hours a night.

Forgo the late night movies

Get some rest and you've find you are much more refreshed and able to do everything a lot more efficiently. Lack of rest sets a series of bad chemical reactions in motion leading to increase stress hormones and higher blood pressure. Greater hunger. Weight gain. Need I go on?

The 10 Sleep Myths have been adapted from the NIH Healthy Sleep Guide:

Myth 1: Sleep is a time when your body and brain shut down for rest and relaxation.
No major organ (brain included) or regulatory system in the body shuts down during sleep. Some physiological processes are heightened during sleep, such as, the activity of the pathways in the brain needed for learning and memory.

Myth 2: Getting just 1 hour less sleep per night than necessary will not have any effect on your daytime functioning. You might not feel tired but even slightly less sleep can affect your ability to think clearly and quickly. Cardiovascular health, energy balance and the ability to fight infections can be compromised.

Myth 3: Your body adjusts quickly to different sleep schedules.
Your biological clock sets your alert times, usually daytime. Thus, even if you work the night shift, you will naturally feel sleepy when nighttime comes. Most people can reset their biological clock by 1–2 hours per day at best. It can take more than a week to adjust to a dramatically altered sleep/wake cycle, such as that when traveling to different time zones or switching from the day shift to the night shift.

Myth 4: People need fewer hours of sleep as they get older.
Older people don't need less sleep, but they often *get* less sleep or less restful sleep. Older people usually spend less time in deep sleep and are more easily awakened. They are more likely to have insomnia or other medical conditions that disrupt their sleep and usually exercise less. Exercise helps promote deep sleep.

Myth 5: Extra sleep at night can cure you of problems with excessive daytime fatigue.
Quality of sleep is as important as quantity. Even with 8 or 9 hours of sleep, you can feel tired because of poor quality sleep. Sleep disorders and/or other medical conditions can affect sleep quality. However, these can be treated effectively with changes in behavior or with medical therapies.

Myth 6: You can make up for lost sleep during the week by sleeping more on the weekends.
Although this sleeping pattern will help relieve part of a sleep debt, it will not completely make up for the lack of sleep. This pattern also will not make up for impaired performance during the week and can affect your biological clock so that it is much harder to go to sleep at the right time on Sunday nights and get up early on Monday mornings.

Myth 7: Naps are a waste of time.
Although naps are no substitute for a good night's sleep, they can be restorative and help counter some of the impaired performance from

lack of sleep. Naps can actually help you learn how to do certain tasks quicker. A couple of tips: avoid taking naps later than 3 p.m. and limit your naps to no longer than 1 hour. If you take frequent naps during the day, you may have a sleep disorder that should be treated.

Myth 8: Snoring is a normal part of sleep.
Snoring during sleep is common. Evidence is growing that snoring on a regular basis disrupts nighttime sleep, making you drowsy during the day and susceptible to diabetes and heart disease. Some studies link frequent snoring to problem behavior and poorer school achievement in children. Loud, frequent snoring can also be a sign of sleep apnea, a serious sleep disorder that should be treated.

Myth 9: Children who don't get enough sleep at night will show signs of sleepiness during the day.
Unlike adults, children who don't get enough sleep at night typically become more active than normal during the day. They also show difficulty paying attention and behaving properly. Consequently, they may be misdiagnosed as having attention deficit hyperactivity.

Myth 10: The main cause of insomnia is worry.
Worry or stress might cause a short bout of insomnia. Persistent insomnia can be caused by: (a) Certain medications and sleep disorders, (b) depression, (c) anxiety disorders, (d) asthma, (e) arthritis, or other medical conditions with symptoms that become more troublesome at night. Some people who have chronic insomnia also appear to be more restless than normal, so it is harder for them to fall asleep. Check the pineal gland, adrenal glands, hypothalamus, pituitary and the liver for good function and health. If that doesn't help, the following tips should also help.

Tips for getting a good night's sleep
-Stick to a sleep schedule. Go to bed and wake up the same time each day.
-Exercise is great but not too late in the day. Try to exercise at least 30 minutes on most days but no later than 5 or 6 hrs before your bedtime.
-Avoid caffeine and nicotine. Coffee, colas, certain teas, and chocolate contain stimulants. They can take up to 8 hours to wear

off. Therefore, any of these after about 2pm can disrupt your sleep. Nicotine often causes smokers to sleep only very lightly. In addition, smokers may wake up too early in the morning because of nicotine withdrawal.

-Avoid alcoholic drinks before bed. An alcoholic "nightcap" doesn't really help you sleep: it robs you of deep and REM sleep, which is needed to feel rested. You also tend to wake up in the middle of the night when the effects of the alcohol have worn off.

-Avoid large meals and beverages late at night. A large meal can cause indigestion that interferes with sleep. Drinking too many fluids too late can have you running to the bathroom all night.

-If possible, avoid medicines that delay or disrupt your sleep. Some commonly prescribed heart, blood pressure, or asthma medications, as well as some over-the-counter and herbal remedies for coughs, colds, or allergies, can disrupt sleep patterns because they contain stimulants. If you have trouble sleeping, talk to your doctor or pharmacist to see if any drugs you're taking might be contributing to your insomnia.

-Don't take naps after 3 p.m. Naps can help make up for lost sleep, but late afternoon naps can make it harder to fall asleep at night.

-Relax before bed. Don't over-schedule your day so that no time is left for unwinding. A relaxing activity, such as reading, listening to music, or listening to a relaxing guided meditation should be part of your bedtime ritual.

-Take a hot bath before bed. The drop in body temperature after getting out of the bath may help you feel sleepy, and the bath can help you relax and slow down so you're more ready to sleep.

-Have a good sleeping environment. Get rid of anything that might distract you from sleep, such as noises, bright lights, an uncomfortable bed, or warm temperatures. You sleep better if the temperature in your bedroom is kept on the cool side. A TV or computer in the bedroom can be a distraction and deprive you of needed sleep. Having a comfortable mattress and pillow can help promote a good night's sleep.

-Have the right sunlight exposure. Daylight helps regulate daily sleep patterns. If possible, go outside in natural sunlight for at least 30 minutes daily. Also, wake up with the sun or use very bright lights in the morning. It is often recommended to get an hour of exposure to morning sunlight to help nighttime sleep.

-Don't lie in bed awake. If you find yourself still awake after more than 20 minutes, get up (yes, stand up) and do some relaxing activity until you feel sleepy. The anxiety of not being able to sleep can make it harder to fall asleep.

If you often find yourself feeling tired or poorly rested during the day despite spending enough time in bed at night, you may have a sleep disorder or an adrenal issue.

photo by Tambako The Jaguar, 2012

Exercise is your secret weapon

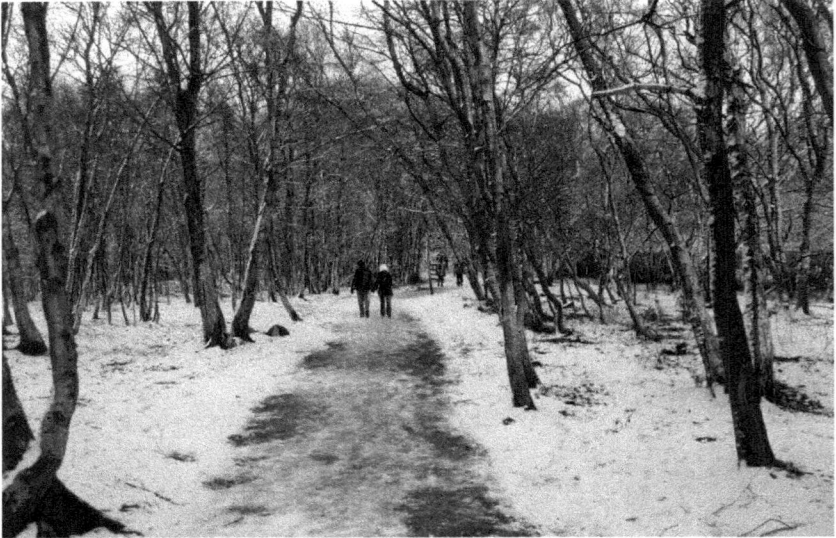

Exercise is a much-ignored aspect of good health. A lot of diet programs will even talk about how their program works even without exercise. Ignore those. There are several reasons why you want to exercise:

It is good for your heart, it lowers cholesterol and blood pressure naturally, and stabilizes blood sugar.

It is good for your brain, it oxygenates it and clears up the brain fog from sitting around too much.

It is better than taking an anti-depressant for relieving dark moods (a brand new study shows this).

It promotes the growth of lean weight or muscle, which

keeps your bones strong and healthy. Plus the more lean weight you have, the better your brain functions.

A good sweat producing exercise releases endorphins and other substances that make your skin look younger.

It dissipates the stress hormones.

Exercise IS Good But How Much Do I Need?

No, you don't have to quit your day job to get enough exercise to be healthy. In fact, research shows that even as little as 30 minutes a day of moderate to vigorous physical activity can help you. What type of activities should you consider? Think about walking, jogging, biking or even gardening. If you're so inclined, join a gym to do the classes like yoga, use the courts, swim, or weight lifting/ cardio machines, preferably the former.

If you haven't been exercising lately, it's very important that you start slowly. Not only that, but before you even begin, double check with your doctor. He'll evaluate your cardiovascular health to see how your system actually reacts to exercise.

Here are some general guidelines you can follow once you make the decision to exercise and prepare yourself with all the preliminaries:

In the beginning, select a form of physical activity that you can participate in for 10 to 20 minutes at a time at a moderate intensity. Good initial choices including walking, biking or even some type of exercise machine at a low speed.

While we've already mentioned that moderate exercise is best, you need to be aware that you need to spend a little time doing it. The American Heart Association recommends that you work your way up to 30 minutes daily. If you're also trying to lose weight, that organization also suggests you get as much as 60 minutes every day.

While that may sound like an extended period of time, you can always break this hour up into 10-minute increments and still reap the profits. Do anything that is fun, enjoyable and that you'll do regularly. For example, take breaks during the day and walk for ten minutes. Better than just choosing one activity, choose several different exercises. In this way you can switch from one to another and not get bored.

Yoga is a great way to unwind and lower stress levels.

Yoga uses a series of exercises and poses, called asanas, that help you relax as well as tone your muscles in order to massage the internal organs. Some yoga practices stimulate all twelve meridians and systems in the body to bring about a feeling of balance and wellbeing. The breathing techniques, called pranayamas, taught in this discipline help to regulate your body's energy levels.

Postures in this practice that promote relaxation also perform the double duty of reducing stress, tension and anxiety. And yoga is a marvelous tool to help improve the flow of your blood and oxygen throughout your body. This rids your system of toxins and other waste.

There's only one catch to the marvelous benefits of yoga. For it to work its apparent magic, you need to perform it on a regular basis. This is not a hit or miss exercise program.

If you're truly interested in yoga as a possible tool, you may want to sign up for a class at a local center. The instructor will introduce you to a half dozen or so poses that specifically target blood circulation.

Summary and Homework

Exercise is a proven secret weapon towards better health, but it also improves cardiovascular health, lowers blood pressure, stress, keeps bones strong, improves your appearance and keeps you younger looking.

Action item for this chapter: Take a 15-minute walk every day this week. If that is too much, start with 5 minutes the first day and work your way up to 15. Check with your doctor to make sure it is okay. If you are already exercising, then seek a way to increase the intensity of your exercise. For example, add one-minute runs interspersed with the walks to increase the distance you walk in an allotted time. You can either increase the speed or distances of your walking to get more exercise. Ideally you want ½ hour per day. You don't have to do this all at once. Exercise is cumulative. Take a walk on your lunch break. Walk up and down stairs between periods of sitting at your desk, such as going to the restroom on a different floor from your office.

Isn't it what you eat, not when?

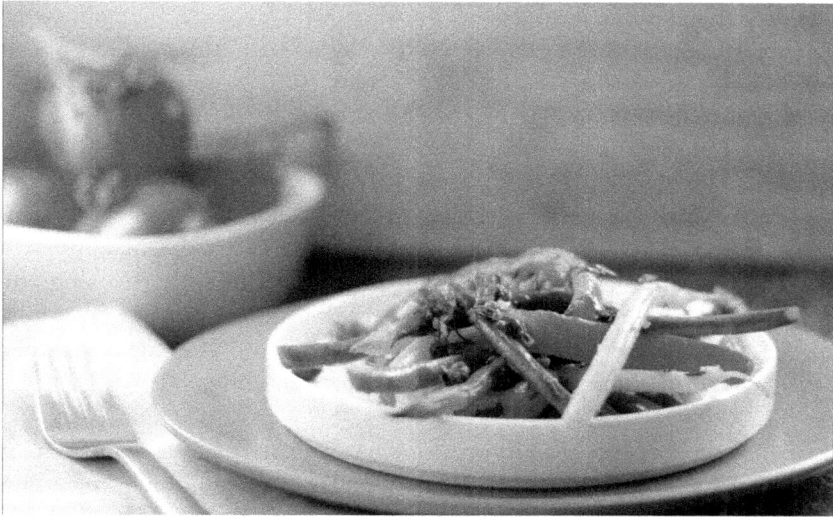

The one concept of healthy eating I resisted for the longest time was increasing my meal frequency. Does this sound familiar? Life was so full, it was hard to imagine fitting in more meals in a day. It turns out that this was self sabotage because eating 4 to 5 to 6 times a day is one of the healthiest things anyone could do, not just for keeping your waist line in check but also for a large number of other health parameters.

In order to keep your blood sugar stabilized, your muscles fed so you can exercise efficiently, and increase your metabolism, you need to eat at least 4 or 5 times a day, but slightly smaller meals. This means the same calories distributed over more meals.

It might sound too inconvenient, hard to fit into a busy, overworked life, and you're thinking: I don't have time to fit all that in. When am I going to eat these meals, fix these meals, when? However, once you try at least 4 meals a day, you may find your mental clarity increased, metabolism increased, fat start to burn off effortlessly, energy levels increased, your days more explosive and no more mid-afternoon slump. You'll find all sorts of time to fit all that into your schedule because you'll have so much more energy.

With four meals a day, you'll also discover that your cholesterol levels get healthier, you'll stop craving food or even being hungry (being hungry is not a good thing despite what anyone says). What a great side effect!

Effect of meal frequency on blood fat levels

The main problem with three bigger meals is that we go for long periods of fasting, blood sugar plummets. Then we eat usually with a larger number of calories, blood sugar rises quickly, causing the insulin levels to go up, thus, converting the blood sugar to fat. This is a major cause of increased blood lipid values. This means higher triglyceride readings and higher cholesterol readings.

Further, this creates a vicious cycle, creating stress due to periods of low blood sugar requiring adrenalin/cortisol to keep going, and then after eating, periods of increased insulin excretion. This is a double whammy, so to speak, with both increased adrenal hormones and increased insulin periodically during each day.

With smaller more frequent meals, blood sugar levels stay steadier, keeping our minds clear (brains need blood sugar to operate efficiently) and our metabolisms going at optimal level. Stress is reduced, insulin is reduced, and fat storage is reduced. Metabolism isn't slowed to help us through a period of too low blood sugar. There is plenty of clinical evidence demonstrating the chemistry of too few meals.

Research found that about half the people eating 3 meals or less a day were not only overweight but had higher cholesterol levels. But only 20% of the people eating 4 or more meals a day were overweight or had high cholesterol levels, a more than statistically significant drop.

Another study measured cholesterol levels in individuals eating three meals a day. When these individuals were fed exactly the same food but in just one meal each day, their cholesterol levels went up. The same food fed as ten meals a day, on the other hand, caused cholesterol levels to fall.

Further studies have shown that grazing, i.e., eating several times a day, not only helps keep cholesterol in check, but can also reduce the levels of other potentially hazardous substances such as sugar, insulin, triglycerides and the stress hormone cortisol. The message is clear: eating less but more frequently offers significant health benefits for the body.

If nothing else, changing meal frequency will have the biggest impact on your health for the least amount of impact on your daily life. If you are already eating healthy, just divide it down and eat smaller meals (or meals and snacks) more often. The bigger the impact, the easier it is to implement. Between eating more frequently and taking a walk every day (next chapter), these may be the two easiest things to implement that will have an enormous impact on your health.

Action Item for this chapter: Break down your meals a bit. Save some for later by eating deliberate snacks between breakfast and lunch, then lunch and dinner. See if that mid afternoon slump disappears!

Where to Begin?

For most of us, consciously transforming our diet is a daunting task. Indeed, if you were to change everything that needed to be changed immediately, it would be overwhelming. Resentment builds up and all our good intentions go out the window.

But more than that, it probably would be totally ineffective. Few of us can bear that much change in our eating habits overnight. Instead, take it one step at a time.

Taking specific small steps can be quite effective. Once you see these small steps as helping you feel better, you'll be much more receptive to tackling other aspects of your diet as you go along. In the following, there are three basic focuses. The first is fat consumption and types of fat, the second is fiber and last, increased consumption of produce.

Let's Start With The Fats: The Good, Bad, and Ugly

It's true! Your body needs fat to function properly. It is high in energy, but that isn't its most important function. Ever since the United States went on this low fat diet craze, we've seen more obesity, more prescriptions for heart medications, and more memory issues. We have gotten fat as a nation. Isn't it time we got sensible and ate our fats again?

Essential fats are needed for our bodies to function properly, as they are key to our cell walls and hormone production. Every gram of fat contains 9 calories, more than double that of protein and carbohydrates.

But too much of anything isn't healthy. This holds especially true when it comes to fats. And all fats are not created equal. Fats supply the building blocks for the essential hormones that make our bodies function. In fact, supplying the right kinds of fat can help alleviate arthritis, skin problems, keep body fat levels down, and give us a real energy boost. The wrong kind of fat creates the inverse conditions, as well as clog our arteries with plaque.

The usual advice is your overall dietary fat intake should be no more than 35 percent of your diet, which provides a feeling of satiety and supplies you with enough of the fats you need for your cells, hormones, and health. I've seen people do well on more fat but too much means cutting down on other important nutrients. Many medical specialists recommend even going as low as 25 percent, although at this level, your skin may dry up and you may start to feel hungry all the time. And then there are certain cardiologists who insist that a person needs to make an even bigger cut in his fat intake. Perhaps these are the very high-risk patients. Some of us do not do well with fat levels below 25%; you each have to experiment because you need to have a feeling of well being. This isn't about torture; this is about feeling great.

Trying to tell the good guys from the bad guys in the world of fats, though, can be difficult. But you can ease the confusion some by remembering there are two broad categories under which all fats fall: saturated and unsaturated.

Let's Examine Briefly The "Bad" Fat

Saturated fat from grain fed animals is associated with heart and circulatory disease. Found mostly in conventionally raised animal products, such as red meat, poultry, butter, and whole milk, it's implicated in raising your blood cholesterol levels as well as increasing your risk of developing heart disease.

By the way, you'll be doing your body a huge favor by reducing your intake of non-organic saturated fats. It's also been associated with a whole host of other degenerative, aging related diseases. This reads, "reducing" not eliminating. Butter for example contains a whole host of fatty acids that are healthy and not obtainable anywhere else. In Ayurvedic medicine (an Eastern style medicine), clarified butter called ghee is used medicinally. Small amounts of organic butter once in a while aren't going to destroy your health

Not all saturated fats are "bad". Coconut oil is also high in saturated fats but is now being sold as "health food" because it is inordinately stable at high temperatures and suitable for cooking. It supplies short and medium chain fatty acids, which do not affect cholesterol levels but are in fact good for you. It has proven to be helpful for those on fat reducing diets. It has NO cholesterol and tastes great when making certain foods. Not all saturated fats are equal!

You can recognize saturated fat immediately. At room temperature they solidify. Think of bacon fat. I remember how my mother used to fry bacon, then save the fat for later use! While it was hot, she'd pour it in a container. When it cooled to room temperature, it was solid. Lard – and even butter – are examples of this type of fat.

Just for the record, many health experts say that saturated fats should make up no more than 10 percent of your total calories for the day. So, if you eat a 2,000-calorie diet, then ideally you should strive to consume no more than 22 grams of saturated fat.

Healthy Unsaturated Fat

There are unsaturated fats that you need to attain optimal health, also known as essential fatty acids or EFAs. Oils and fats are made up of fatty acids. Depending on the type you choose, unsaturated fat can help improve your overall health and lower your risk of developing certain diseases.

And perhaps here is where confusion reigns: because within this broad category of fat, there are several sub-categories. Fatty acids are long chain molecules. They are categorized by: (a) their chain length and (b) the position of any unsaturation along the chain. That is what the 3 and 6 represent in omega-3 and omega-6 fats. It is the position along the chain where you find the "unsaturation". *Unsaturated* means that it doesn't have all the hydrogen it could possibly have. As soon as you add them, you get "hydrogenated fats", the ones created by overheating them, such as those found in margarine and possibly every other "stabilized" fat in foods found on the shelf.

Unsaturated fats fall into two broad categories. Ones with single unsaturation points or <u>monounsaturated</u> oil, and ones with more, called <u>polyunsaturated</u>.

If you look at oil sources and the break down of oils, no source is all one type of fatty acid. Foods are actually a combination of many types of fats or fatty acids. The more unsaturation points an oil has, the lower the solidification temperature. So, saturated fat is solid at room temperature, while olive oil, which is mainly monounsaturated fat, will start to solidify in the refrigerator. However, corn oil, which is polyunsaturated, will require a deep freeze to make it solid.

Good sources of monounsaturated fat include olive and avocado oils. There are several foods that also contain an abundance of this healthy fat, most notably avocados and just about all nuts, especially macadamia nuts.

Good sources for polyunsaturated fats are sunflower or nut oils. These fats are less stable outside of their natural food, particularly at room temperature and in the light. They will break down and go rancid quickly. That is why it is preferable to use monounsaturated fats in salad dressings and so forth. Fats and nuts should be refrigerated so they keep longer and you don't end up eating even partially rancid food.

Omega-3 Fatty Acids: King of Fats

Under the category of polyunsaturated is still one more type of fat. You've undoubtedly heard something about this fatty acid. It's Omega-3. It is the golden ticket to optimal health because it is an essential fatty acid that is the precursor for all the good things in our bodies.

The source of for this oil is mostly seafood such as cod liver, salmon and tuna, although you'll find it in a few other foods as well, most notably flax seed. In fact, these essential fatty acids are so important in maintaining your health, that I'm devoting an entire section to this variety of polyunsaturated fat.

For many, however, getting to 35 or 25 percent intake is a great start, you can decide once you get that far how much lower you need to go.

As you might guess, you'll want to keep your consumption of fats to as much as possible of the good kind. These include vegetable fats, normally called monounsaturated and polyunsaturated fats. And you'll want to include Omega-3 fatty acids, much of which come from fish. Lemon flavored cod liver oil goes down pretty easily and keeps in the frig for a good month.

Many fish and seafood products contain omega-3s but they are a two edged sword. Many also contain high levels of mercury.

In summary, the goal is to increase the good fats, especially omega-3s and monounsaturated fats and decrease saturated fat from animal products. Again as mentioned in an earlier chapter, eliminate trans fatty acids and canola oil all together.

Increase Your Fiber Consumption

Fiber comes in two forms, <u>soluble</u>, meaning it dissolves in water, and <u>insoluble</u>. While both fibers are excellent additions to your diet, increase the amount of soluble fiber you consume daily as this has been proven to reduce cholesterol and improve health.

Fiber is found in abundance in fruits, vegetables, legumes, and whole grains (not refined white flour or sugar!). Rich sources of soluble fiber include rolled or whole oats, oat bran, brown rice and psyllium husks in the grain category; apples, plums, oranges and tangerines in fruits; broccoli, carrots, peas, potatoes, summer squashes including zucchini in vegetables; and pinto beans in legumes. You see a lot of really delicious foods are in this category.

A note of caution however, processing some foods, such as brown rice cakes, most cold cereals, instant oatmeals, and some freeze drying processes break down the fiber so it is less effective. Choose whole fresh food rather than processed and slow cooking instead of instant to get the most fiber.

But Your Body Doesn't Digest Fiber!

As important as it is to your health, you may be surprised to learn that your body can't break down this compound. Because it isn't digested, your body does not really absorb it.

Fruits and vegetables are great sources of fiber, naturally, as are whole grain produces like breads and cereals. In addition, you'll find fiber in nuts and legumes, another term for beans and peas of all kinds!

For a substance your body doesn't absorb, it's of great benefit to your health. Not only does it improve your intestinal health, fiber also helps to prevent heart disease and possibly some cancers.

You'll discover that most foods contain some combination of both insoluble and soluble fiber. The fiber actually speeds the movement of food through your intestines. This promotes regularity and bowel health.

Fiber, by the way, is usually excreted for the most part intact. Insoluble fiber is found in whole-grain foods like wheat bran as well as many vegetables and fruits with the skin still on it. Soluble fiber, by contrast, dissolves when you mix it with water. You might hear this referred to as viscous fiber. Then it becomes a gel-like substance. It actually slows the transit of food through the small intestine.

How Much Fiber Do You Need?

The National Academy of Sciences says that men up to age 50 need a minimum of 38 grams of fiber daily. Women in this age group need a minimum of 25 grams. For men who are older than 50, it's highly suggested that they receive 30 grams daily. Women in this same age group are encouraged to eat at least 21 grams daily.

We've already mentioned how to increase your fiber content. But it definitely bears repeating. Eat more fruits, vegetables and legumes. While you're increasing your consumption of these foods, you should take the opportunity right now to decrease your consumption of packaged and processed foods. I know I've mentioned this before, but it really is that important!

Dietary changes summary
1. Keep fat consumption between ~25 - 35% of your calories
2. Eliminate trans-fatty acids (partially hydrogenated), (soy, peanut also recommended), and non-food fats such as canola oil.
3. Reduce saturated fats from non-organic animal sources.
4. Increase unsaturated fat consumption, particular omega-3
5. Increase fiber intake, especially soluble fiber.

Action steps:

Take an omega-3 supplement daily. Add a source of soluble fiber such as Metamucil or psyllium husks and eat more fruits, vegetables and unprocessed grains such as brown rice if you're not allergic. Cut down on saturated fats from non-organic sources.

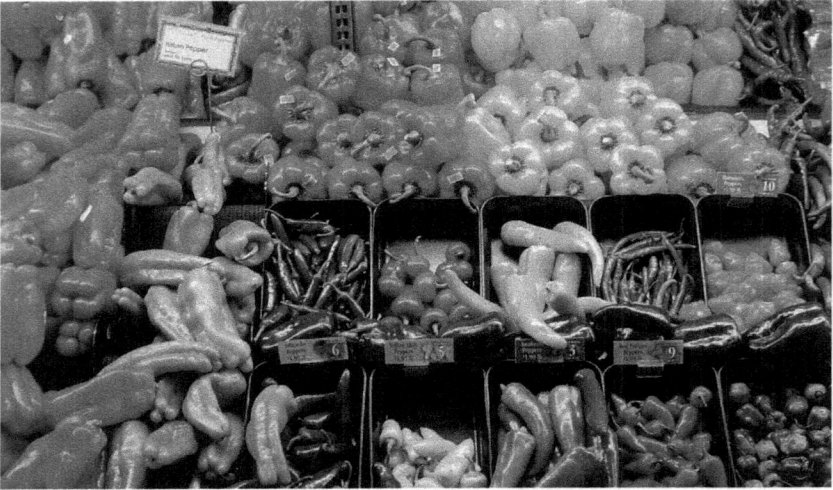

Basic healthy diet:

1.   This baseline diet template is very balanced and health-oriented. The calories can be adjusted from fat loss to muscle gain depending on your goals. Include a variety of natural foods, including   complex carbohydrates, fruits, low or non-fat dairy products, and lean proteins.   It is not vegetarian or vegan based, which is a whole other book unto itself.   This is a simple place to start.   The most important is to get as much fresh and even raw produce as possible.   This promotes health and reduces inflammation (if you are not allergic to it).

2.   Eat smaller, frequent meals. Eat approximately every 3 to 4 hrs.   The earlier meals may be larger than evening meals. The last meal of the day should be light and if possible, eaten two to three hours before going to sleep.

3.   You can mix or match proteins for any time of the day.   You can also mix or match fruit and veggies (and dairy if okay) for any time of the day.

4.   Essential fats go well with your protein and green vegetable

meals. Avoid eating fats with large amounts of carbs for best weight control.

5.   Use spices and flavorings generously to season your food to make it more interesting and palatable. You can add any low or non-caloric condiments and sauces such as low calorie marinades, salsa, cinnamon and other spices. You can also use a wide variety of herbs, spices and seasonings such as pepper, garlic powder, oregano, parsley, sage, thyme, dill, ginger, chopped onion, paprika, Mrs. Dash, and any no-sodium seasoning mix. If you use salt, use sea salt, preferable Himalayan or Celtic.

6.   There's no need to avoid eating at restaurants; you just need to know what to ask for. You must carefully read menus, learn how to make sensible selections, ask about how your food is prepared. Pay very close attention to portion sizes and extra calories from butter, oils and sauces are frequently added, but not noticed.

7.   Almost all restaurants accommodate healthier eaters and even those of us with food allergies. Almost all of them have gluten free menus, for example. Even fast food restaurants now have salad bars, low calorie dressings, and gluten free selections.

You can get a template for tracking food (recommended for a week or two until you pass through some adjustment period) by visiting http://scientifichealer.com/book-bonus/ and sign up with your email.

Sample meal structure: see the definition of the descriptions below.
7 am Breakfast:
      Lean Protein 2 to 4 oz, Starchy carb (3/4 to 1 c.) or simple carb, any fibrous carb,
10 am snack (optional):
      Lean Protein 3-6 oz, Starchy carb (3/4 to 1 c.) or simple carb, any fibrous carb.
1 pm Lunch:
      Lean Protein 3-6 oz, Starchy carb (~1/2 c. or none), Fibrous carb (vegetable/salad)
4 pm Snack (optional):
      Lean Protein 3-6 oz., Fibrous carb (vegetable/salad), essential fat

7 pm Dinner:
Lean Protein 3-6 oz, Fibrous carb (vegetable/salad), essential fat.

Food groups
Complex Carbohydrates: (Fibrous)
- Asparagus
- Cauliflower
- Peas
- Collard greens
- Lettuce
- Tomatoes, pasta sauce, salsa
- Broccoli
- Green Beans
- Cucumber
- Mushrooms
- Salads
- Spinach
- Okra
- Brussel Sprouts
- Squash
- Zucchini
- Pepper, green or red
- Kale

Natural Simple Carbohydrates (Fruit)
- Apples
- Bananas
- Berries
- Grapes
- Grapefruit
- Unsweetened applesauce
- Oranges
- Nectarines
- Peaches
- Pears
- Blueberries
- Raspberries
- Plums
- Cantaloupe

- Pineapple
- Mango
- Papaya
- Jelly (all fruit)

Complex Carbohydrates (Starchy)
- Potatoes (white, red)
- Yams, sweet potatoes, carrots, plantains
- Beans, lentils, legumes
- Note: get organic as much as possible
- whole grains, Note: while okay for some people, are usually best left alone if you are recovering from some health issue or have an autoimmune problem. Try quinoa or buckwheat, which are both not grasses but flowers.

Lean Proteins:
- Chicken breast,
- Turkey breast
- Fish (Flounder, Haddock, Salmon, Orange Roughy, Cod, Tuna etc.)
- Shellfish (Lobster, shrimp, Clams, etc.)
- Lean Red Meat (Flank Steak, Round Steak, extra lean sirloin)
- Eggs/Egg whites (One yolk for every six whites)
- Organic dairy products (milk, cheese, yogurt, cottage cheese, etc.)
- Note, again go for grass fed organic foods. Many of the animals are fed GMO corn and grains and the effects will carry through to the flesh of what you're eating.

Dairy Products (if not allergic, grass fed organic best, the fatty acid ratios improve)
- Milk
- Cheese
- Yogurt
- Cottage cheese
- Note, go for dairy made from grass fed beef, all organic otherwise the grain they're fed will come through.
- Caution again on dairy, it is allergenic for many people and if you have an autoimmune problem, go through a period of avoidance.

Fats
- Nuts & seeds,
- flaxseed oil,
- olive oil, extra virgin only,
- olives,
- fish fat
- organic butter or ghee
- Avocados,
- Coconut oil/fat, get the best quality, organic and extra virgin

1.   How to structure your day:

A typical set of meals are easy to fit into any day. Schedule
    7am – Breakfast
    10am – Snack #1 (optional)
    1pm – Lunch
    3pm – Snack #2 (optional)
    6pm – Dinner

The following sample menus are suggestions. You can substitute any vegetable, meat and fats into the basic structure. You can use either a fruit or a portion of carbs at meals and snacks until 3 pm.

7 am:

Breakfast:

Protein Choices:

Choose One
    2 whole organic eggs
    2 oz organic chicken, beef, or turkey
    2 oz of leftover meat from the night before

Vegetable Choices: Choose One
    1 cup cooked broccoli
    1 cup cooked cauliflower
    1 cup sautéed spinach
    1 cup steamed asparagus

Fat Choices: Choose One
    1/4 Avocado
    2 teaspoons flax seed oil (do not cook with flaxseed oil)
    2 teaspoons extra virgin olive oil

Examples:
        2 eggs
    1 cup steamed cauliflower

2 tsp flaxseed oil over the cauliflower

2 oz. chicken
1 cup spinach
1/4 Avocado

2 oz. beef
1 cup cooked broccoli
2 tsp extra virgin olive oil

Snack #1 (10-11am) and Snack #2 (3-4pm)
Protein Choices:
Choose One
    2 TBSP Natural, Raw Almond Butter
    1 oz Raw Almonds 1 oz Raw Walnuts
    1 oz Macadamia nuts
    1 oz Raw Pecans
    2 hard boiled eggs
    2 oz turkey (dark or white) or chicken (dark or white)
Vegetable Choices:
Choose One
    Celery Sticks
    10 Baby Carrots
    1 sliced red, yellow, or green pepper
    1 large sliced tomato
    2 cups broccoli or cauliflower
Examples:
    1 oz raw almonds
    1 large sliced tomato

    2 hard boiled eggs
    1 yellow pepper

    1 ounce raw macadamia nuts
    10 baby carrots

Lunch (1-2pm) and Dinner (6-7pm)
Protein Choices:
Choose One
4 ounces chicken (dark or white meat)

4 ounces turkey (dark or white meat)
4 ounces fish or seafood (tuna only 1 time per week)
3 ounces beef (lean varieties)
Over a large salad that is made up of any of the following: All lettuce except for Iceberg (It has no nutritional value)
Celery, Peppers, Cucumbers, Tomatoes
Vegetable Choices: Choose One
1 cup cooked broccoli
1 cup cooked cauliflower
1 cup sautéed spinach
1 cup steamed string beans
1 cup sauteed zucchini or other summer squash
1 cup steamed bell peppers
1 cup cooked asparagus

Examples:
4 oz grilled chicken (white or dark)
Over a large salad made up of Romaine lettuce, tomatoes, cucumbers and celery
1 cup asparagus added to the salad or on the side
Bragg Organic Apple Cider Vinegar and 1 Tbsp flaxseed oil as dressing

Or
3 oz beef burger
Over sautéed spinach
Salad on the side with Bragg Organic Apple Cider Vinegar and
1 Tbsp extra virgin olive oil

Carb Choices:
Choose One
1/2 cup cooked brown rice
1/2 cup cooked millet
1/2 cup cooked quinoa
1/2 cup or 4 oz cooked sweet potato
1/2 cup cooked beans (any variety)
Fruit Choices:
Choose One
1/2 green apple

1/2 pear
1/4 medium banana
1/2 cup berries (strawberries, blueberries, raspberries, blackberries)
1/2 cup fresh pineapple

By regulating the portions and calories, if your weight doesn't come down to a good place automatically, you can lose fat relatively easily.

11. Twenty-six rapid stress busters

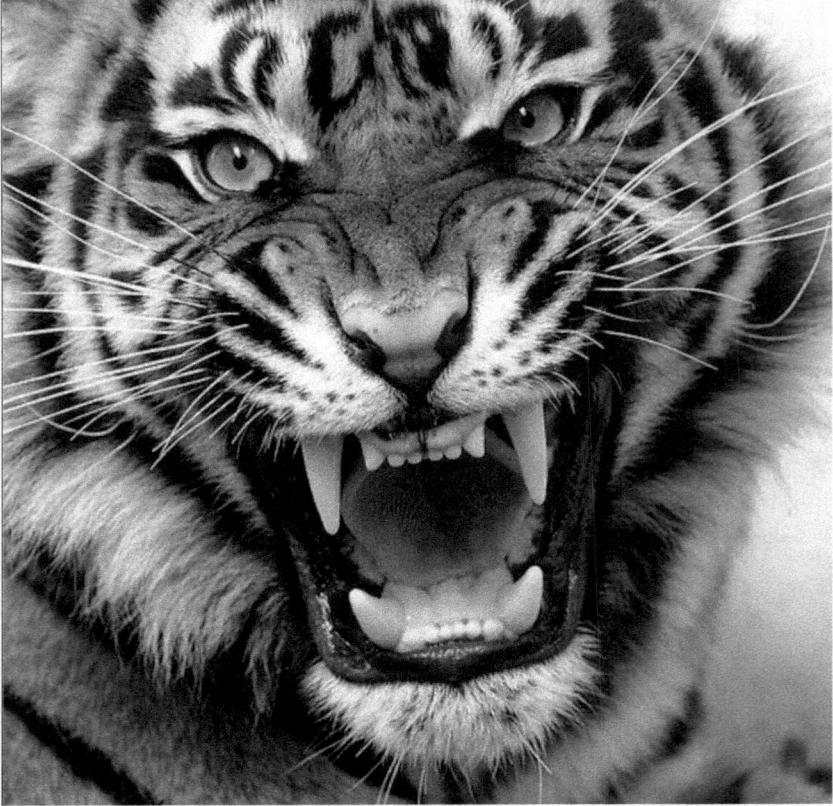

"Reality is the leading cause of stress amongst those in touch with it."
Jane Wagner

As mentioned in Chapter 2, there are eight factors important for maintaining vibrant health—seven of them are more important than food.

Many of these factors are mentioned throughout the chapters of this book. For those in my classes or those that have seen me speak, I pass around what I call an abundance wheel as shown in the figure. Ideally the wheel should be full, so it is symmetric and relatively full. If one of those areas are too low (we fill them in from the inside out at each section), to show you exactly what area of your life needs the most help. You can go ahead and try a muscle test on what your values are and where you need to go.

Scientific Healer
Abunance Wheel

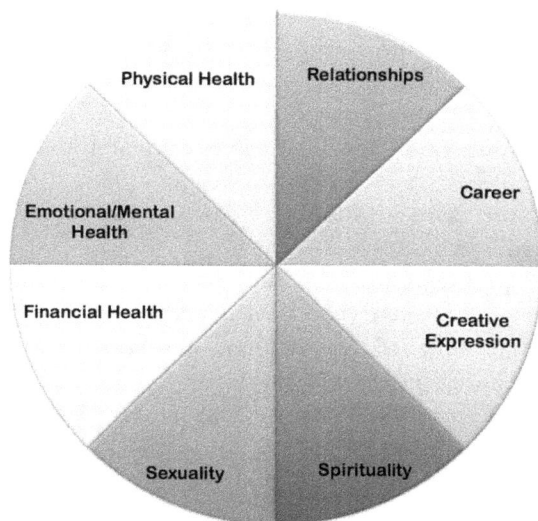

Here are the brief descriptions of each of the sections:

1. **Relationships**: Are your relationships loving and nurturing or critical, negative or draining. This includes your relationship to yourself. Do you have a strong inner voice critic that makes you wrong or not good enough?

2. **Career**- Is your career fulfilling and satisfying or is it something you drag yourself every day to just to pay your bills. Is there some way you can transform it as LeAnn did?

3. **Creative Expression**: Express yourself in some art form or other, whether it's art, music, poetry, prose, acting, decorating, etc.

4. **Spirituality**: having a connection to a higher power and using it in daily life.

5. **Sexuality**: having a deep connection with another human and expressing that love.
6. **Financial health:** Not necessarily wealth, just a good relationship with your wealth and wealth management.
7. **Emotional/mental Health:** Balanced emotionally and mentally.
8. **Physical health**: Having a good diet, exercise, rest, hydration – the foundations of good physical health.

Many of the ideas of how to get unstressed mentioned throughout this book will help you fill the sections that are lacking. If you've never taken the emotional stress assessment, here's your opportunity to see where you stand. This test has been around for decades.

How do you know you are stressed: take the stress questionnaire?
Common symptoms of stress include having a fuzzy memory, where you can't remember even your best friend's name or why you stood up from a chair to go do something. A second is that you have a lightheaded feeling when you stand up. The adrenal glands are overworked. A third would be that no matter how much sleep you get, you have no oomph.

Life Stress Questionnaire – Each life change has a number associated with it that indicates the average stress toll this event takes on people. Each person is different but it will give you a clue if you are emotionally stressed.

Have you had any of the following things happen to you during the past year? Jot down the numbers following each of the events you've experienced, and add them up to get your grand total.

Life Event	Point Value
Change in social activities	15
Change in sleeping habits	15
Change in residence	20
Change in work hours	20
Change in church activities	20
Tension at work	25

Small children in the home	25
Change in living conditions	25
Outstanding personal achievement	30
Problem teenager(s) in the home	30
Trouble with in-laws	30
Difficulties with peer group	30
Son or daughter leaving home	30
Change in responsibilities at work	30
Taking on major financial responsibility	30
Foreclosure of mortgage or loan	30
Change in relationship with spouse	35
Change to different line of work	35
Loss of a close friend	35
Gain of a new family member	40
Sexual difficulties	40
Pregnancy	40
Change in health of family member	45
Retirement	45
Loss of job	50
Change in quality of religious faith	50
Marriage	50
Personal injury or illness	50
Loss of self-confidence	60
Death of a close family member	60
Injury to reputation	60
Trouble with the law	65
Marital separation	65
Divorce	75
Death of a spouse	100

Grand total	_____

Your total score measures the amount of stress to which you have been subjected. A score of 150 or less is just about the normal level most of us deal with on an ongoing basis. With a score of 150 to 250, you're seriously stressed and most likely are experiencing the effects of toxic stress. If you scored 250 to 300, you're clearly in a stress-overload situation. Above a score of 350, you are seriously stressed and need to take action now. If your score is over 350, you might consider seeking professional help through this difficult time in your life.

26 Stress Busters That Anyone Can Do

The thought of doing one more thing to those of you that are overwhelmed can be, well, overwhelming. But believe it or not, mustering up the energy to try one or two of these stress busters can help calm that feeling of overwhelm.

1. Have more fun. Take time to do things that are pleasurable, even if it is only for a few minutes a day. This might be to sit down and listen to some music, draw a picture, enjoy a hobby, take a hot bath, get a massage, buy something new, talk to a friend or sit outside with a cup of tea or coffee with someone that you enjoy. We forget to take time out for ourselves when everything is so pressing. Doing this helps us get our minds off the thinking that makes us so stressed in the first place.

2. Human touch is healing and soothing. Hug a family member or friend. When I was very ill, I asked my young children to give me 3 hugs a day to help me get better. They felt better and I felt better. We would laugh about it if it got to be close to bedtime and they still needed another hug. If that isn't possible or comfortable, getting a massage, haircut or manicure also helps because of the individual pampering you are getting.

3. Humor. Laughter really reduces the stress hormones in your system and boosts your immune system through increasing the natural killer t-cells. Find the humor in life, watch funny movies, go to see comedians you enjoy. Read jokes. Read Irma Bombeck, Andy Rooney or Dave Barry.

Read the morning comics or a "Far Side" collection. You'll find that once you see the lighter side of life and learn to laugh more, things just won't seem so dire.

4.   Meditate, even if only ten minutes a day. You can go to my website http://diamondhealingmethod.com to get an 13 minute audio that calms and soothes for free. Meditation lowers cortisol and brings the body into the parasympathetic state.

5.   Improve your posture. Yes, stand up straighter, taller, and stop hunching over. Recent studies have shown your body language can either put your body into a stressed or relaxed state. Hunching over is stress inducing while standing up straight raises testosterone and reduces adrenaline and cortisol.

6.   A healthy eating plan will improve your health and your resiliency. It will fuel your body with the things it needs to rejuvenate and restore itself.

7.   Exercise is particularly relaxing, it is known to reduce blood pressure, bad cholesterol, and stress hormones, such as cortisol. Getting up and walking, stretching, and deep breathing are simple ways to de-stress. It can also include yoga, gardening, swimming, going to the gym, cycling or anything else that gets the body going.

8.   Breathe deeply, slowly, and deliberately to help your body relax.

9.   Music. Most people respond well to music. Did you know that conductors are amongst the longest lived occupations? They are active, standing and directing the music, but also listen intently to it. Singing is a huge stress reliever, particularly if you push the air up using the abdominal muscles. It promotes deep breathing and forces you to concentrate on something other than worries. Play an instrument.

10.   Remove yourself from your daily environment. Are you running from home to work to the store to the doctor to the store to work to home, etc? This puts you on an endless treadmill. Go somewhere in nature, a park, a beach, a forest, a mountain, somewhere out of the way of your normal routine, if only to just sit and look or to walk/run/hike. Go alone or with a friend (not someone that stresses you).

Breaking up the daily routine with a mini-vacation will most certainly help you cope with stress.

11. Get enough sleep. Lack of sleep raises cortisol levels, makes you hungrier, and takes you out of healing mode and into survival mode.

12. Focus on gratitude. Instead of bemoaning some event, find something positive that came out of it. For instance, after I divorced my husband, which was a terrible and stressful event in my life, I forgave him with gratitude. I was grateful I had these two beautiful children in my life. I was grateful I had a good career in research. I was grateful for things he taught me and the good years we had together. Releasing the anger and tension helped me lower my levels of stress. Every event has a lesson somewhere even if it is unpleasant. You gain strength and wisdom through challenges and difficulties. Find out what they are.

13. Don't procrastinate. Pay your bills when they arrive, make your appointments immediately, throw out your junk mail when it arrives, finish your assignments as soon as possible, don't wait until a deadline looms until tackling something. Having something finished and taken care of releases your mind from having to cope with all the stress of thinking about what you need to take care of. Even prepare things ahead of time, such as planning what you will wear, eat, and do the next day. This makes it clear.

14. Keep your life as simple as possible. Don't buy and accumulate a lot of stuff. We need a lot less than we think we do. Give it away, sell it, donate it. Don't keep clothes you don't wear, books you don't read, computers you don't use, programs you don't use, and dishes you don't use. Keep your environment as orderly as possible. A clean environment is a great deal less stressful.

15. Keep lists and a calendar. This way you have your tasks ahead of you and checking them off the list is a way to relieve the stress of one more thing that has been accomplished.

16. Keep your life as honest as possible. Telling lies, cheating, and stealing are stressful. It also dims your light. The fear of being caught is not worth whatever it is. Did you know that people have been fired from superb jobs for cheating on

their travel vouchers? A hundred dollar lie caused them to lose 5 and 6 figure incomes. It is so not worth it, is it?

17. Find ways to keep out of stressful situations. Here are some of my stress savers: there's a lockbox with a house key near my front door, a spare car key in my purse, and spare change in the car for parking. Allow enough time to get to appointments promptly, bring a magazine, a short meditation audio, or a laptop to appointments so there's something useful to do while waiting. Get your car serviced regularly and get regular dental checkups. Don't let your gas gauge go too low. What are yours?

18. Learn to say "no" to people and things. Neither their world nor yours will be affected by the "no" but you will feel less stress. This includes unplugging your phone or turning the ringer off, deciding you don't absolutely have to do all the things you set out to do (prioritize), the world won't end if you don't get to the vacuuming today, for example. Become more flexible; rigidity and trying to control everything is stressful.

19. Make your ringtone, alarm tone, and doorbell soft and gentle so it doesn't jangle you.

20. Write a journal for five to fifteen minutes every morning. Putting thoughts down on paper will help the whirlwind mind calm down. It works.

21. Talk with someone you trust. Just say everything you need to say, but don't always come back to the same story then. Do something about whatever is bothering you.

22. Socialize, go to get-togethers or throw one yourself, with some help if you need to. Throw a potluck with some friends or meet at a nearby restaurant.

23. Live one day at a time and do one thing at a time. Decide on a task and do that one thing. Don't hop from one thing to the next, doing them all poorly.

24. Don't put yourself down. Instead make a list of your attributes. We are our own worst critics and the constant flow of criticism gets in the way of enjoying life. Your circumstances don't matter. Liking yourself has nothing to do with your circumstances. Go improve your appearance: buy a new article of clothing, shoes, get your hair or makeup done, get a manicure.

25. Volunteer. Doing something for someone less fortunate than we are reminds us of how lucky we really are. No matter how bad our circumstances are, there are those that are much worse off. Whatever it is, as long as you take good care of your health, you can survive it.
26. Affirmations are one of the best ways to turn stress into a positive force in your life. Say affirmations in the present as if they have already occurred. "Something wonderful is happening today, I can just feel it." "I think, am, and feel rich."

Stress takes its toll on our well being, quality of life and health. A direct correlation exists between stress and illness and early death.

Summary

Stress is unavoidable in you life. Good coping mechanisms include taking care of issues before they become a problem, looking at events in new ways and stress releasing techniques. Without them, healing your stress will not effect permanent change. Healing the stress includes taking care of the spiritual, emotional and mental effects that are either causing stress or a result of stress. Then finally, your physical body is healed of these effects. Without altering the response to stress, health problems would eventually return. Remember, your natural state is one of joy and happiness. Don't let stress take that away.

Exercise

Once a day, stand up straight with hands on hips and feet shoulder width apart. It looks like you're standing like Superman or Wonder Woman. Stand like this for two minutes a day and while doing this, think of three things that you can be grateful for while taking deep relaxing breaths. This lowers your cortisol (the major stress hormone) by 20% and raises your testosterone by a similar amount. It doesn't take long and can diffuse potential muscle spasming or other signs of physical stress.

Appendix I: Improving energy systems in the body

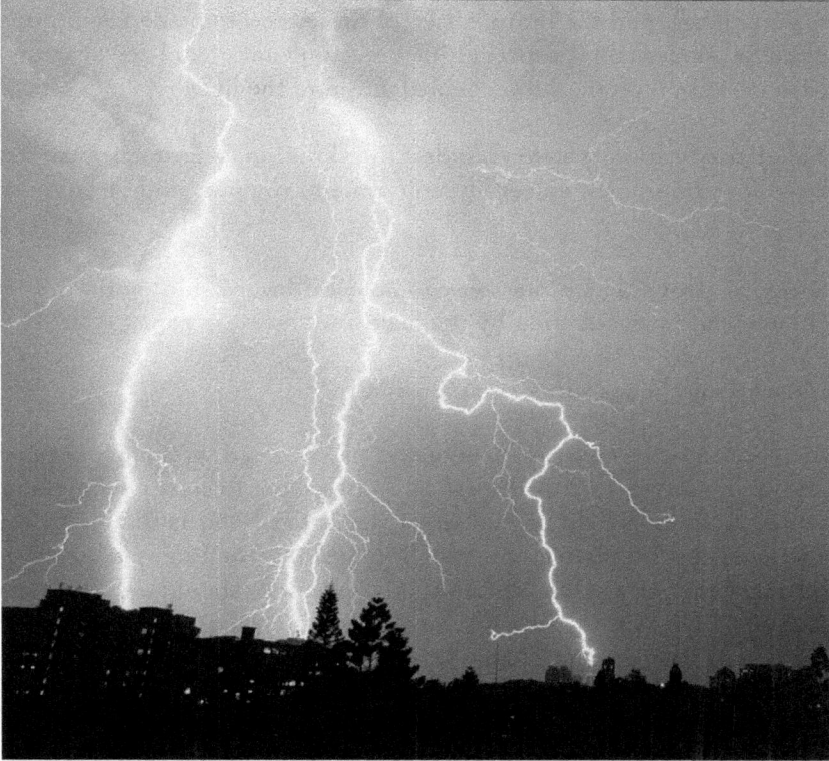

"Each moment of worry, anxiety or stress represents a lack of faith in miracles, for they never cease."
T. F. Hodge

The glands and organs in your body keep you energized and detoxified.

Your body has redundant systems that keep you fed/energized, detoxified, safe, and allow you to reproduce. Some of our organs or glands do double or triple duty and there are some redundancies.

The glands and organs involved in energy production are:

Tongue, nose, stomach, pancreas, adrenal glands, thyroid, liver, gall bladder, small intestine, hypothalamus, pituitary, lungs, circulatory system, heart, and the brain. Two of these tend to be depleted quite often in modern life, especially if you don't take care to clear and replenish them often, the adrenal glands and the liver.

The detoxification system includes: the skin, lungs, kidneys, bladder, large intestine, liver, spleen, lymph system, thymus, and circulatory system.

Safety is provided by the senses, muscles, brain, skin, and adrenal glands while reproduction by the male and female organs.

Muscles and bones support our structure.

As you can see, energy production is involved in many organs/ glands in our body. It is helpful to know where to start when you or someone seeking help complains of being tired and is unable to get adequate rest no matter how much they sleep, for example. Going through the processes outlined in this book should get systems energized quickly. In reality, once you're proficient, clearing and energizing the energy channels and fields, the emotions, and the brain will take a only matter of 10 to 20 minutes. The explanation of the process and the physics behind it takes much longer. The intent is the most important aspect of the Diamond Method, not the exact process. This process works very well but it isn't the only one that does. It does cover all aspects of our existence. As one client said, I no longer have to go to five different practitioners to help me get well.

How do your energy systems fail?

Exhaustion is a very common problem in modern society. If you compare it to how a human's life was even a hundred or two hundred years ago, it's vastly different in terms of pace. Even my own work in the laboratory: before computers, I just stood at the instruments and watched the chart come off, marked the chart, matching the dial to the position of the pen, and it took its time.

After computers were connected to the instruments, I could leave the room and multitask. No time for mental rest. It's the same everywhere. We try to get more and more done in less and less time, even to the point of multitasking and doing nothing well.

I'm sure every one of you can identify.
1. Fast pacing: We are electronically connected 24/7 and usually are multi-tasking. Conducting business while exercising or flying on a plane, helping children with their homework while cooking, and dictating into a recorder while driving are common multitasking jobs. We feel like we have to because there is way too much to do and only 24 hours in a day to do it. In the 1950s, it was rare to have a working mother, now it is the rule and not the exception.
2. Sudden stimuli: Phones ringing, horns honking, city noise, sirens, nearby dogs barking, people living in close proximity, long travel times to and from work, all jangle our nerves and leave us little time to simply "be" and quietly regenerate. We stuff so much in a day because we demand it and not because we have to. We try to have it all when a re-evaluation of this should take place.
3. The modern workday: We usually start at some time early in the morning, and go through the day, coming home in the evening with little time during the day to rejuvenate. In some countries, the siesta style workday is still in place, such as Spain or Greece, where everything closes down between 1 and 5 pm in the day and people go home to rest then arrive back at work later in the evening and stay up late. Sleep is in shifts, basically, where stress levels are fundamentally reduced. In the United States and many industrialized countries, the old way of rejuvenating after a time of working is not possible if we want to hold a regular job.
4. Nourishment and environmental toxins: If our bodies are working overtime to detox without enough healthy nourishment for rebuilding, our energy systems have no way to rejuvenate and replenish.
5. Lack of restful sleep: Too many people who want it all sleep in a too noisy house in a too bright city. Converting your sleeping space into a more serene, darker, and soothing environment will help your systems get restored.

When your energy is down, here's where to start.

If, after clearing the energy channels and fields, centering the spirit in the body, clearing and healing the brain, raising the life force and lowering the toxicity and inflammation in the body, you still don't have energy and mental clarity back, there are a number of systems in the body to look at more closely. As mentioned in a previous section of this chapter, the body has several redundant systems that have to do with energy. The places to look are:
1. Low grade infections.
2. Adrenal exhaustion.
3. Liver dysfunction.
4. Hypothyroidism (low thyroid function)
5. Mitochondrial problems/converting to energy.
6. Digestive malfunction, e.g., celiac's disease or food allergies (see Chapter 8).
7. Autoimmune issues.

These supplements may help with your energy:

1. Omega-3 fatty acids, such as fish oil, 1 - 2 capsules or 1 - 2 tbs. of oil daily, to help decrease inflammation and help with immunity. Omega-3 fatty acids may increase the risk of bleeding, especially if you already take blood-thinning medication. Ask your doctor before taking omega-3 fatty acids if you take blood thinners such as warfarin (Coumadin) or if you have a bleeding disorder.
2. L-tyrosine, 500 mg two to three times daily. The thyroid gland combines tyrosine and iodine to make thyroid hormone. If you are taking prescription thyroid hormone medication, you should never take L-tyrosine without direction from your doctor. Do not take L-tyrosine if you have high blood pressure or have symptoms of mania. On the other hand, L-tyrosine is a good booster of energy and brings a feeling of "normalness" from a fatigue you may have been feeling.
3. L-Carnitine, 2 gm daily, 1 morning, 1 evening. It is also an energy booster as it aids the liver in supplying energy to the muscles and boosts memory as it helps supply the brain glycogen.
4. Eleuthero or Siberian ginseng - it has a healing and slightly stimulating effect.

Here are two of the most important glands in your body for energy: the adrenal glands and the thyroid.

Alleviate exhaustion by repairing these two small glands.

Your adrenal glands are two small glands that sit atop your kidneys, which are located on each side of your spine about an inch above your waistline. They are chiefly responsible for releasing hormones in response to stimuli or stress through the synthesis of corticosteroids such as cortisol and catecholamines such as adrenaline (epinephrine) and noradrenaline. These endocrine glands also produce androgens in their innermost cortical layer. The adrenal glands affect kidney function through the secretion of aldosterone. In today's society, you are being bombarded by stimuli that cause our adrenal glands to secrete hormones: bells and phones chiming, alarm bells, car horns, loud noises, jack hammers, tires screeching, people arguing, dogs barking, cats screeching, etc. It's a cacophony of sounds that can drive your adrenal glands into overdrive. These stimuli release the stress hormones and send your body into a reactionary state known as the sympathetic state. In this condition, your body is being prepared to run from the proverbial saber tooth tiger. But, wait, there isn't a tiger hiding around the corner. It was just the phone that sent your blood pressure sky high. It takes about half an hour to come back down to the calm state known as the parasympathetic state in which our bodies are renewing themselves. By constant stimuli all day long, the adrenal glands can get exhausted.

Some adrenal conditions, such as Addison's disease, show up in the same way. In either case, the protocol is the same.

Adrenal glands tend to store feelings of overwhelm and worthlessness. A healthy color for the adrenal glands is a caramel brown, which is really a darker version of orange, a happy color. Unhealthy colors are black, brown, white and gray.

Fight or Flight — The Stress Response

Nobel Prize winner Dr. Hans Selye, the father of stress research, proposed three stages to this stress response. This "General Adaptation Syndrome" (GAS) consists of alarm, adaptation, and finally, exhaustion. His model is useful in helping you see where you are in the stress cycle and what to do about it.

Alarm Stage

When you are first stressed, in the *alarm* phase, the brain signals your adrenal glands to pump stress hormones into your bloodstream. There are about forty such hormones, but the most important stress hormones are adrenaline, which is manufactured by the inner core; cortisol; and DHEA (dehydroepiandrosterone). Cortisol and DHEA are produced by the outer shell, or *cortex*.

Both adrenaline and cortisol give a boost to your blood sugar, which gives you the energy to run from danger. The adrenal glands also release the hormone DHEA, which helps maintain energy and resistance to stress.

As a result of this rapid deployment of adrenaline, cortisol, and DHEA, we have more oxygen and sugar available, push more blood to the brain and muscles, and are instantly more alert. In fact, many people will create stress in their lives just to experience this stimulation. It may be stress, but it's also a high.

Adaptation Stage

When the body needs to continue its defense mechanism beyond the initial "fight or flight" response, it enters the *adaptation* phase. Cortisol and DHEA have a reciprocal relationship, so as cortisol levels go up, DHEA levels fall. We start to feel the effects of long-term stress, with increasing anxiety, fatigue, and mood swings.

Exhaustion Stage

When we become stuck in the stress response, it becomes chronic, and we enter the dangerous territory of the *exhaustion* phase. No longer can we produce the necessary cortisol to respond to stress. Our DHEA levels drop. We become depleted of vitamins, including vitamin C, the B vitamins, and essential minerals such as magnesium. Our energy plummets, and since adrenaline is derived from the "feel-good" neurotransmitter dopamine, excess adrenaline demands lead to dopamine deficiency. Consequently, our emotions can take a dive into depression.

The outer part of the adrenal gland, the cortex, makes the following:
Cortisol, the stress hormone
DHEA, an energizing hormone that declines with age, hence the decline in energy with age
Aldosterone, the hormone that maintains salt and water balance in your body

Estrogen and **testosterone**, the primary sex hormones, are also produced in small amounts by the adrenal glands.

Even though your body is designed to return to normal after stress, many of us are under continuous stress, keeping cortisol levels consistently high. This eventually leads to adrenal fatigue. Although this condition affects millions of people, conventional medical practitioners are still skeptical about its existence and won't treat adrenal weakness until the glands are in full collapse, called Addison's disease.

Testing the adrenal glands

Take the Adrenal Stress Index laboratory test to discover if you are suffering from toxic stress. It involves a series of samples over the course of a day to measure your DHEA and cortisol levels.

Here are the DHEA normal ranges (saliva):
Women ages 19–30: 29–781 mcg/dL
Women ages 31–50: 12–379 mcg/dL
Postmenopausal women: 30–260 mcg/dL

And the cortisol normal ranges:
Morning: 4.3–22.4 mcg/dL
Night: 3.1–16.7 mcg/dL

If your test results are outside the normal ranges, you are certainly suffering from stress overload, and the many ways of alleviating your stress will give you relief. Normal is highly relative, and these scores are a bit deceptive. The important points are that DHEA diminishes with age and that cortisol should be higher in the morning than at night. The "normals" you deal with will be your own.

You might want to consider retaking the lab test for stress at the end of an eight-week cycle of following the guidelines in this book to see how you are doing. Your results will be clearly explained in the report that accompanies your test results.

Self-Test for Adrenal Fatigue
Here's an excellent self-test for low adrenal function. You'll need a blood pressure cuff or monitor and a helper.

Lie on your back for at least five minutes. Then have your helper record your blood pressure.

Sit up quickly and have your blood pressure taken again.

Stand up quickly and take it again.

In people without adrenal dysfunction, the blood pressure will rise between 4 and 10 points with each measurement. If your blood pressure drops for either or both of the last two measurements, it's likely that you have adrenal exhaustion.
****

One of the most important glands in your body is the thyroid gland.

Few people really know or understand thyroid deficiency even though it is a common problem and can affect their health in profound ways. Most people are not aware of what their thyroid does, where it is, and how it can affect health. In fact, more than half the people with thyroid deficiency are undiagnosed and probably a good percentage of those that have are on the wrong doses of thyroid hormone to be physically at their peak.

What is the thyroid is what does it do?

The thyroid is a gland that sits at the base of your neck right above the clavicle. It is a butterfly shaped gland and it can get swollen if it is not working properly (this is called a goiter). The hormones it produces, mainly T3 and T4, but also T1 and T2, regulate metabolism or the speed of chemical reactions in your body, from head to toe. Every cell in your body has a thyroid receptor. If you don't have enough thyroid hormone, all processes will slow down.

Food absorption slows, making getting nutrition and energy from food difficult, leads to malnutrition, constipation, and fatigue. Sometimes the skin can turn orange from inadequate metabolizing of beta-carotene.
The immune system is depressed, leading to increased infections and illness, lack of resistance, and increased inflammation, which is one of the big factors in heart and arterial disease.
The healing processes slow, skin lesions and injuries take much longer to heal. Premature aging, dry and cracking skin, slow hair and nail growth, dry brittle hair, and loss of hair can occur.

Current estimates put thyroid deficiency or hypothyroidism at about 4.6% of the population, but I suspect this may be higher because (a) the current guidelines for testing are unable to diagnose sub-clinical cases easily and (b) many people are simply not routinely tested unless they complain of an obvious set of hypothyroid symptoms. See suggestions for testing below.

Symptoms of low thyroid function or hypothyroidism

The trouble with diagnosing hypothyroidism is that many other problems have similar symptoms. For example, aside from the obvious turning orange or having a goiter (check your neck to see if it looks swollen at the base), many of the symptoms can appear as depression or a number of other age-related problems. Taken as a whole however, they can point to a thyroid problem. In any case, thyroid deficiency should be tested for. The most common symptoms include:

- Weight gain or inability to lose weight even on a low calorie diet
- Fatigue, exhaustion
- Cold extremities even if it is warm out
- Low body temperature
- Depression, anxiety
- Constipation
- Poor short-term memory, slowed speech
- Menstrual irregularities
- Dry coarse and thinning hair
- Dry cracking skin
- Muscle pain, joint pain, carpal tunnel syndrome, tendonitis
- High blood pressure, high cholesterol

These symptoms should prompt you to ask for a thyroid test. Since many doctors do not do a thorough testing (including testing for individual thyroid hormones), let the following be your guidelines. But first it is important to realize how your diagnosis can be missed.

What does it mean if I have subclinical hypothyroidism.

A subclinical case is one in which the patient suffers symptoms but the lab slip declares them healthy. There are several reasons why this can occur: the main one being that many testing labs have not yet converted their values to the 2003 standards for the main diagnostic hormone, which is called TSH or thyroid stimulating hormone. TSH comes from the pituitary and tells the thyroid gland to release more hormone if blood levels of thyroid hormone are low.

The lower the TSH, the more responsive the thyroid gland is to releasing enough thyroid hormones. Most people feel their best at a level of about 1 mIU/L. The old "healthy" levels were up to 4.5 or even 5.5 mIU/L. In 2003, these were lowered to 2.5 or 3 mIU/L depending on the lab doing the testing. However, one of the biggest testing labs still uses the old values. For, example at a TSH level of 3.5 mIU/L, my hair was literally falling out by the handfuls and my skin was so dry it cracked. Other people are not so affected.

Another reason why a TSH value might be in range but a patient might suffer from hypothyroidism is that of the thyroid hormones T3 is metabolically active, while T4 is produced by the thyroid gland. The body (in the liver mainly) must convert the T4 to T3 and if that process isn't efficient, then there is inadequate T3 to rev up the metabolism.

The way to discover this "defect" is to have both free T3 and free T4 levels tested. The healthy free T3 range is 2.3 to 4.2 pg/mL and for free T4 0.8 to 1.8 ng/L. While a range is given, most people feel at their best when their values are balanced to the median level within this range. An extreme to either end, while not necessarily wrong for any one patient, might not quite be right if symptoms persist.

Table: Range of Healthy Values for Thyroid Tests

Hormone	Range	Optimal
TSH	0.5 - 2.5 mIU/L	1.0mIU/L
Free T3	2.3 - 4.2 pg/mL	~3.2 pg/mL
Free T4	0.8-1.8 ng/L	~1.3 ng/L
Thyroid Antibodies*		
Thyroglobulin	<20 IU/mL	<20 IU/mL
Thyroid Peroxidase	<35 IU/mL	<35 IU/mL
*Varies by lab		

What thyroid tests should I get?

Many doctors, even excellent doctors, don't always understand the interplay between these three hormones. One should have not only TSH tested, but also free T3 and free T4, and possibly thyroid antibodies to test for an autoimmune problem such as Hashimoto's.

There are a series of nutritional tips that may help alleviate the symptoms or even the cause:
1. Eat foods high in B-vitamins and iron, fresh vegetables, and sea vegetables.
2. Avoid foods that interfere with thyroid function: these are called goitregens as they interfere with iodine absorption or inhibit other thyroid functions. Eat these cooked as it

helps neutralize the problem. These include broccoli, cabbage, Brussels sprouts, cauliflower, kale, spinach, turnips, soybeans, peanuts, linseed, pine nuts, millet, cassava, and mustard greens. Kale and broccoli are milder.

3. Go gluten free and even grain free. Go with whole fresh foods and not processed. The Paleo Diet is a good one to follow to help heal your thyroid and even bring it back to healthy functioning.

4. If you take thyroid hormone medication, talk to your doctor before eating soy products. There is some evidence soy may interfere with absorption of thyroid hormone.

5. Taking iron supplements may interfere with the absorption of thyroid hormone medication, so ask your doctor before taking iron.

6. Eat foods high in antioxidants, including fruits (such as blueberries, cherries, and tomatoes) and vegetables (such as squash and bell pepper).

7. Avoid alcohol and tobacco. Talk to your doctor before increasing your caffeine intake, as caffeine impacts several conditions and medications.

8. Do not take an iodine supplement unless your doctor tells you to. Iodine is only effective when hypothyroidism is caused by iodine deficiency, which is rare in the developed world. And too much iodine can actually cause hypothyroidism.

9. Filter your shower water with a chlorine filter if your water is chlorinated because you will take the chlorine in through your lungs as the water is atomized in the shower. Chlorine blocks thyroid entry into your cells slowing down your metabolism needlessly.

Appendix II: Brief Summary of Protocols

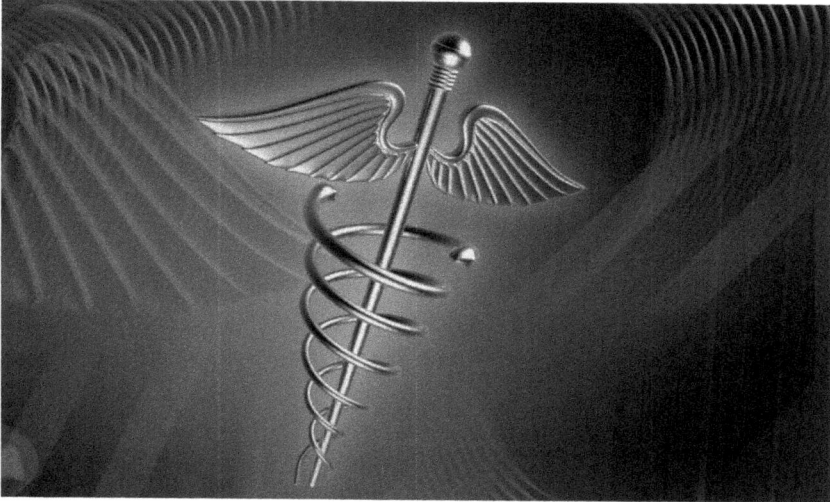

The healing protocols are scattered throughout this book. Here is a brief summary if you have no idea where to start:

1. The first thing you do is develop your own yes-no test: Chapter 4

2. With your yes-no test, measure how open your seven major portals are. I use a scale from 0 to 100. See Chapter 3 for what each of the major chakras or portals feed, emotionally, mentally and physically. It will give you a clue as to where you are depleted. Open them up to allow them to feed you again. You can use the motions described in Chapter 3 or whatever you are comfortable with. It's intent that's important.

3. Measure the energy of the 5 major portions of your brain. Chapter 6. Boost the energy of those areas lacking. Anything below 70% energy is needed some real healing. The method of doing this is mentioned in Chapter 8. Bring the master cell of that area up to full energy and tell the rest of the cells to copy it.

4. Check life force, which is how well your spirit is attached to your

body.   If it's low, boost it up by sending healing energy to it.

5. Check how well your body can heal. As you get older, your body usually thinks it can't be at 100% health. It's a myth. That myth needs dispelling. Shoot healing energy into that idea to dissipate the myth.

6. Check the toxicity levels in your body. If they're high, dissipate the toxic molecules with healing energy.   Drink plenty of filtered water and eat as much clean organic food as possible.   The more produce the better, especially vegetables, raw nuts, and seeds, such as walnuts, chia or flax seeds.

7. Check the inflammation levels in the body, dissipate them with healing energy. The nourishment instructions in number 6 are good for inflammation, too.

8. Check how centered your spirit is in your body. If it is off center, bring it back to center with healing energy.

9.   Now the question will be, "is my next step a.   Spiritual, b. Emotional, c. Mental, or d. Physical?"   Once you've ascertained that, you go through the processes outlined in this book in the various chapters.   For example, emotional can be a trapped emotion or a relationship issue.   Mental can be a brain healing needed, a brain organ healing, or a mental pattern dictated by family, tribe or community. Spiritual could be a past life issue, the spirit being out of balance with the body, a portal being closed down or a foreign spirit, which we have not covered here.   Physical is healing a gland, organ or system.

Healing the separate glands and organs are beyond the scope of this book as well as detailed discussions of their various functions.   I have written it all down and it turned into a 500+ page book.

10.   Much of the science comes into play in setting the hormonal cycles, the brain chemistry cycles on a function such as a sine wave, filtering out the energy you don't want to reach you with certain filters, detailed programming on the DNA also known as epigenetics (which can also be controlled with diet and behavior) or stem cell

release, which are many of the examples as given in this book. There is much more. The main thing is to experiment both with intent and knowledge. Read about a condition then set the intent to work on it. You are all creators and can create the life and health you envision. If you need help with any of this, please contact me.

Appendix III: Reading list

Recommended reading for the health/healing minded individual.

Alexander, Dr. Eban - Proof of Heaven - Doctor's account of dying and returning to tell this tale. http://scientifichealer.com/proof-of-heaven

H.S. Burr in Wikipedia (http://en.wikipedia.org/wiki/Harold_Saxton_Burr)

Diamond, Dr. John - The Body Doesn't Lie - Applied Kinesiology and universal symbols for humans http://scientifichealer.com/body-doesnt-lie

Gordon, Richard - Quantum Touch: the Power to Heal - another healing modality that has a lot of interesting elements that could be useful to you. http://scientifichealer.com/quantum-touch

Hawkins, Dr. David - Power vs. Force - introduces a scale of emotions and verifies the usefulness and accuracy of applied kinesiology. http://scientifichealer.com/power-vs-force

Malarkey, Kevin and Alex - The Boy Who Came Back from Heaven: A Remarkable Account of Miracles, Angels, and Life beyond This World While some of this account is fabricated by a little boy who wanted to please his family, some of it was not. This was a miraculous healing of a child that should have died. http://scientifichealer.com/boy-who-came-back-heaven

Myss, Carolyn - Anatomy of the Spirit - unifying principles of religions and how the dis ease of the spirit leads to the dis ease of the body. scientifichealer.com/anatomy-spirit

Nelson, Dr. Bradley - The Emotion Code - methodical discovery of how emotions affect your health and recovery http://scientifichealer.com/emotion-code

Northrup, Dr. Christiane - Women's Bodies, Women's Wisdom - treatise on women's coming of age into their wise years. http://scientifichealer.com/womens-bodies-wisdom

Orloff, Dr. Judith - Second Sight - Journey of awakening http://scientifichealer.com/second-sight

Pert, Dr. Candace - The Molecules of Emotion - ground breaking book on the discovery of the endorphin receptors and the first indication that Eastern healing had a physical basis. http://scientifichealer.com/molecules-emotion

Stilbal, Vianna - Theta Healing: Introducing an Extraordinary Energy Healing Modality - a different twist on energy healing: many elements are interesting and usable no matter what the modality http://scientifichealer.com/theta-healing

Who is Anastasia?

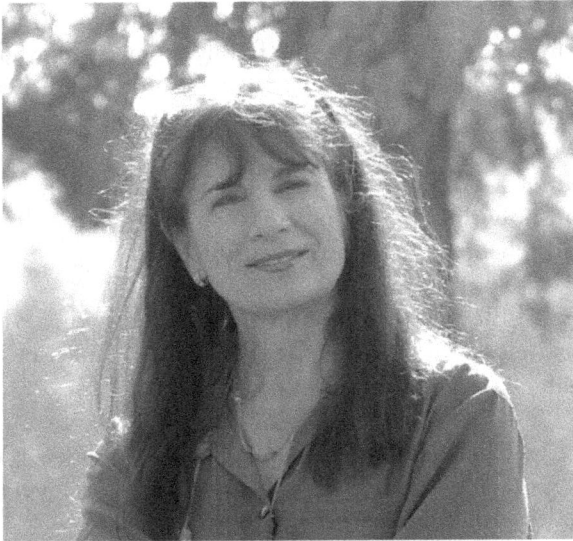

Dr. Anastasia Chopelas, the Scientific Healer, is the founder of the Diamond Method, a sophisticated healing technique that includes molecular and vibrational healing, nutrition, herbal medicine, fitness, and lifestyle.

After completing a Masters degree in Geochemistry at Caltech, Dr. Chopelas graduated from UCLA with a PhD in Chemistry. She spent the following thirty-eight years in geophysical research at prestigious institutions, including the Max Planck Institute for Chemistry in Mainz, Germany; University of Nevada, Las Vegas; University of Washington; and UCLA where she also contributed chapters in numerous books and published articles that have since become the genesis for courses.

It was while studying mineral vibrations at extreme conditions and the properties inherent in them, that Anastasia became aware of her gift . . . the ability to psychically tune into the cellular, emotional and physical levels of *human beings*. Soon after this realization, she began to dive into the esoteric sciences.

After she became a Reiki Master 20 years ago, Dr. Chopelas studied psychic phenomenon, shiatsu, reflexology, and acupressure to heal emotional distress, physical dis-ease, and spiritual unrest.

Understanding quantum mechanics helped Anastasia see how healing energy permeates time, dimension, and space. Her knowledge of chemistry allowed her to envision and create healing starting at the molecular level.

Now, blazing a new trail via The Diamond Method, Anastasia has helped hundreds of people move out of dis-ease and has written the book: "Get Rid of Bad Cholesterol," practical guides for regaining your health and getting off medications.

Anastasia lives in Torrance, CA., where she has a private practice and travels extensively teaching people how to maintain and sustain healing long term. She has founded the Scientific Healer's Academy to teach her methods.

Schedule a complimentary 20 minute discovery session at http://scientifichealer.com/appointment/. If you are interested in setting up a healing appointment or having Anastasia speak to your group or center, please call: 310-692-4036 or contact http://scientifichealer.com/contact/

More from Dr. Anastasia Chopelas

Live Seminars, Tele-classes, and Online Courses. Contact Anastasia at 310-692-4036 or http://scientifichealer.com/contact/ Anastasia teaches you how to heal yourself, the energy systems of the body, and how to live your best life. Check her website, http://scientifichealer.com for live seminars. To book her to speak, Contact her at the phone number or contact at her website.

Listen to Anastasia on Diamond Healing Radio soon to be Scientific Healing with Dr. Anastasia Chopelas on Vivid Life Radio. Visit scientifichealer.com/radio/ or download from iTunes https://itunes.apple.com/us/podcast/diamond-healing-radio/id939276568?mt=2

CHOPELAS

www.ingramcontent.com/pod-product-compliance
Lightning Source LLC
Chambersburg PA
CBHW070902270326
41927CB00011B/2434